Chronic Fatigue Syndrome

How You Can Benefit from Diet, Vitamins, Minerals, Herbs, Exercise, and Other Natural Methods

Chronic Fatigue Syndrome

How You Can Benefit from Diet, Vitamins, Minerals, Herbs, Exercise, and Other Natural Methods

Michael T. Murray, N.D.

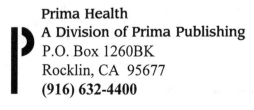

Prima Health
A Division of Prima Publishing
P.O. Box 1260BK
Rocklin, CA 95677
(916) 632-4400

PRIMA HEALTH and colophon are trademarks of Prima Communications, Inc.

Library of Congress Cataloging-in-Publication Data

Murray, Michael T.
    Chronic fatigue syndrome : how you can benefit from diet, vitamins, minerals, herbs, exercise, and other natural methods / Michael T. Murray.
        p.   cm. — (Getting well naturally series)
    Includes bibliographical references and index.
    ISBN 1-55958-490-4
    1. Chronic fatigue syndrome. 2. Naturopathy. I. Title. II. Series.
RB150.F37M87   1994
616'.047—dc20
                                                                94-7471
                                                                CIP

        99 00 01 AA 10 9
Printed in the United States of America

How to order: Single copies may be ordered from Prima Publishing, P.O. Box 1260BK, Rocklin, CA 95677; telephone (916) 632-4400. Quantity discounts are also available. On your letterhead, include information concerning the intended use of the books and the number of books you wish to purchase.

Visit us online at www.primahealth.com

Contents

SECTION *III* *Addressing the Causes of Chronic Fatigue* 115

11 Plant-Based Medicines for Chronic Fatigue   159

SECTION *IV* *Putting It All Together*   171

12 The Energy Prescription   173

Preface

Have you ever experienced an abundance of natural energy running through your body and mind? If you did, how did the world look to you? Was everything brighter? Did the challenges of your life seem less significant? How did you relate to the people around you? How did you feel about yourself and the people you love?

Vibrant natural energy is truly a wonderful feeling that too few people experience on a consistent basis. The number of Americans suffering from fatigue is staggering. Fatigue is the most common medical complaint in medical practice. It is also a complaint that the current medical system has very little answers for. Fortunately, a new medical model is emerging that focuses on health rather than disease.

It is my hope in writing this book that the reader will follow the guidelines and recommendations presented to live a more energetic and passionate life. I know the recommendations work—I have seen them work in my own life, the lives of my patients, and the lives of my friends and family members.

Although the book focuses on the chronic fatigue syndrome, a newly defined syndrome linked to low immune function and chronic viral illness, the answers provided are appropriate for anyone seeking higher energy levels. Practical information is provided so that the recommendations given can easily be utilized.

This book is not based on theory, it is based on firm rational scientific and medical ground. The recommendations given throughout the book are designed to improve your whole being—your mind, body, emotional state, physiology, and, of course, your energy level. More and more, there is a greater appreciation for the interconnectedness of the mind and body as well as the individual body systems.

Chronic fatigue syndrome may be the prime example of a "general system failure." It seems to affect every body function, especially the immune system and the mind. In turn, these two body systems are influenced tremendously by the environment, internal physiology, nutritional status, and other factors.

The approach presented in this book may be the most comprehensive approach for chronic fatigue syndrome and chronic fatigue ever written. I have read many books on these subjects, including many medical textbooks, but they always seemed to be missing something. In the case of chronic fatigue, nothing can be overlooked.

By reading this book, I feel extremely confident that my hope will be realized—that you, the reader, will experience greater vitality and passion in your life.

Acknowledgments

The major blessings in my life are my family and friends. My love for them truly makes life worth living.

Special appreciations to my wife, Gina, for being the answer to so many of my dreams; to my parents, Cliff and

Patty Murray, and my grandmother, Pauline Shier, for a strong foundation and a lifetime of good memories; to Bob and Kathy Bunton for their love and acceptance; to Ben Dominitz and everyone at Prima for their commitment and support of my work; to Terry Lemerond and everyone at Enzymatic Therapy for all of their friendship and support over the years; to Joseph Pizzorno and the students and faculty at Bastyr College who have given me encouragement and support; and finally, I am eternally grateful to all the researchers, physicians, and scientists who over the years have strived to better understand the use of natural medicines. Without their work, this series would not exist, and medical progress would halt.

Michael T. Murray, N.D.
April 1994

Before You Read On

- Do not self-diagnose. Proper medical care is critical to good health. If you have symptoms suggestive of an illness, please consult a physician—preferably a naturopath, holistic physician or osteopath, chiropractor, or other natural health care specialist.
- If you are currently taking a prescription medication, you absolutely must consult your doctor before discontinuing it.
- If you wish to try the natural approach, discuss it with your physician. Since he or she is most likely unaware of the natural alternatives available, you may need to do some educating. Bring this book along with you to the doctor's office. The natural alternatives being recommended are based upon published studies in medical journals. Key references are provided if your physician wants additional information.
- Remember, although many natural alternatives, such as nutritional supplements and plant-based medicines, are effective on their own, they work even better if they are part of a comprehensive natural treatment plan that focuses on diet and lifestyle.

Chronic Fatigue Syndrome: An Overview

1

What Is Chronic Fatigue Syndrome?

C hronic fatigue syndrome (CFS) is a newly established name that describes a persistent and varying combination of symptoms including recurrent sore throat, low-grade fever, lymph node swelling, headache, muscle and joint pain, intestinal discomfort, emotional distress, depression, and loss of concentration.

Although newly defined and currently prevalent, CFS is not a new disease. References in the medical literature to a similar condition go back as far as the 1860s. Since then, chronic fatigue syndrome has been known by a variety of names including chronic mononucleosis-like syndrome or chronic EBV syndrome, Yuppie flu, postviral fatigue syndrome, postinfectious neuromyasthenia, chronic fatigue and immune dysfunction syndrome (CFIDS), Iceland disease, Royal Free Hospital disease, and many others. In addition, symptoms of chronic fatigue syndrome can mirror symptoms of neurasthenia, a condition first described in 1869.

Chronic fatigue syndrome was formally defined in 1988 by a consensus panel convened by the Centers for Disease

Control (CDC) because guidelines for evaluating patients with chronic fatigue of unknown cause were needed by clinical physicians and researchers.[1] In response, a formal set of diagnostic criteria was established by the CDC. But these criteria have been controversial. For example, psychological symptoms are both a minor criterion and a potential grounds for denying a diagnosis of CFS. One major complaint from physicians is that the CDC definition is better suited for research than for clinical purposes. Also, the CDC criteria ignore many common symptoms noted by patients diagnosed with CFS (see Table 1.1).

CDC Diagnostic Criteria for Chronic Fatigue Syndrome

Major Criteria

New onset of fatigue causing 50% reduction in activity for at least six months

Exclusion of other illnesses that can cause fatigue (discussed in Chapter 2)

Minor Criteria

Presence of 8 of the 11 symptoms listed or 6 of the 11 symptoms and 2 of the 3 signs

Symptoms

1. Mild fever
2. Recurrent sore throat
3. Painful lymph nodes
4. Muscle weakness
5. Muscle pain
6. Prolonged fatigue after exercise

Table 1.1   Frequency of Symptoms in CFS

Symptom/Sign	Frequency (%)
Chronic fatigue	100
Low-grade fever	60–95
Muscle pain	20–95
Sleep disturbance	15–90
Impaired mental function	50–85
Depression	70–85
Headache	35–85
Allergies	55–80
Sore throat	50–75
Anxiety	50–70
Muscle weakness	40–70
Prolonged fatigue after exercise	50–60
Premenstrual syndrome (women)	50–60
Stiffness	50–60
Visual blurring	50–60
Nausea	50–60
Dizziness	30–50
Joint pain	40–50
Dry eyes and mouth	30–40
Diarrhea	30–40
Cough	30–40
Decreased appetite	30–40
Night sweats	30–40
Painful lymph nodes	30–40

7. Recurrent headache
8. Migratory joint pain
9. Neurological or psychological complaints
   Sensitivity to bright light
   Forgetfulness
   Confusion
   Inability to concentrate

Excessive irritability

Depression

10. Sleep disturbance (hypersomnia or insomnia)
11. Sudden onset of symptom complex

Signs

1. Low-grade fever
2. Nonexudative pharyngitis
3. Palpable or tender lymph nodes

You may find that you do not meet the strict CDC criteria necessary to be formally diagnosed with CFS. Whatever your symptoms, the recommendations and guidelines in this book will help improve your energy level and regain your vitality.

British and Australian criteria for diagnosis of CFS are less strict than the CDC's.[2] The minor criteria are not absolutely required and the major criteria are not as strict. For example, the Australian definition regards as major criteria the onset of fatigue at a level which causes disruption of normal daily activities (in the absence of other medical conditions associated with fatigue).

Using the CDC criteria, the diagnosis of CFS in individuals suffering from chronic fatigue is about 11.5%. Using British criteria about 15% of these individuals qualify, while the Australian criteria apply for about 38% of these patients.[2]

Epstein–Barr Virus and CFS

Many research studies have focused on identifying an infectious agent as the cause of CFS. While still controversial, the Epstein–Barr virus (EBV) has emerged as the leading culprit.[3-7]

EBV is a member of the Herpes group of viruses, which includes Herpes simplex types 1 and 2, Varicella zoster virus,

Cytomegalovirus, and Pseudorabies virus. A common aspect of these viruses is their ability to establish a lifelong latent infection after the initial infection. Latent infections are generally kept in check by a normal immune system, but when the immune system is compromised in any way, these viruses can become active as viral replication and spread. This is commonly observed with Herpes virus infections, especially in immunocompromised individuals such as those with AIDS, cancer, or drug-induced immunosuppression.

Infection with EBV is inevitable among humans. By the end of early adulthood almost everyone will have in their blood detectable antibodies to the Epstein–Barr Virus, indicating past infection. When the primary infection occurs in childhood there are usually no symptoms, but in adolescence or early adulthood, the clinical manifestations of infectious mononucleosis develop in approximately 50% of cases.

Although reports of a prolonged or recurrent mononucleosis-like syndrome began appearing in the 1940s and 1950s, it wasn't until the 1980s that evidence implicated EBV in this broad clinical spectrum of chronic fatigue and associated symptoms. Numerous studies of patients presenting these symptoms have now demonstrated persistently elevated titers (levels) of serum antibodies against the Epstein–Barr Virus (specifically, anti-EBV capsid antibody titers greater than 1:80).

A careful study of 134 patients who had undergone EBV antibody testing because of suspected chronic mononucleosis-like syndrome, found mixed results. Fifteen patients complaining of severe, persistent fatigue of unknown origin were compared with 119 patients with less severe illness and with 30 age- and race-matched controls.[8] The more seriously ill patients generally had higher levels of EBV antibodies than did the comparison groups, and, interestingly, they also demonstrated higher antibody titers to Cytomegalovirus, Herpes simplex viruses types 1 and 2, and measles. This led researchers to conclude, "some patients with these illnesses (syndromes of chronic fatigue) may have an abnormality of infectious and/or immunologic origin," and that there remain "questions concerning the relationship between CFS and EBV."[8]

Current knowledge about EBV infection can be summarized as follows:

1. EBV and the Herpes group of viruses produce latent lifelong infections.
2. The host's immune system (T lymphocytes, interferon, and other lymphokines) normally holds the latent infection in check.
3. Any compromise in the immune system can lead to reactivation of the virus and recurrent infection.
4. The infection itself can compromise and/or disrupt immunity, thereby leading to other diseases.
5. Elevated EBV antibody levels are observed in a significant number of diseases characterized by immunological dysfunction.
6. Elevated antibody titers to the Herpes group viruses, measles, and other viruses have been observed in patients suspected of having CFS and who also display elevated EBV antibody titers.

EBV antibody testing (and antibody testing for other Herpes group viruses and measles) may be useful as a measure of immune function and overall host resistance, but should not be exclusively relied upon for diagnosis of CFS.

In addition to EBV, a number of other viruses have been investigated as possible causes of CFS. This search for a viral agent is consistent with the common current medical approach: to focus on the infectious organism rather than on reducing susceptibility and supporting the individual's immune system to deal with the organism effectively.[3-5]

Organisms Proposed as Causative Agents in CFS

Epstein–Barr virus

Human herpes virus-6

Inoue–Melnich virus

Brucella

Borrelia bugdorferi

Giardia lamblia

Cytomegalovirus

Enterovirus

Retrovirus

Immune System Abnormalities and CFS

There is little argument that a disturbed immune system plays a central role in CFS. A variety of immune system abnormalities have been reported in CFS patients. Perhaps the most consistent abnormality is a decreased number or activity of natural killer (NK) cells.[3,4,9,10] NK cells received their name because of their ability to destroy cells that have become cancerous or infected with viruses. In fact, for a time, CFS was also referred to as low natural killer cell syndrome (LNKS).

Other consistent findings include a reduced ability of lymphocytes, key white blood cells in the battle against viruses, to respond to stimuli.[10] One of the reasons for this lack of response may be reduced activity or decreased production of interferon. Interferon is a special chemical factor produced by the body that acts as a natural protector against viruses. Increasing interferon levels is extremely important in activating the white blood cells to destroy cancer cells and viruses. Both low and high levels of interferon have been reported in CFS, but in most of the cases interferon levels are depressed. When interferon levels are low, reactivation of latent viral infection is likely. Conversely, when interferon (as well as other chemical mediators like interleukin-1) levels are high, many of the symptoms may be related to interferon. When interferon is used as a therapy in cancer and viral hepatitis, the side effects it produces are quite similar to the symptoms of CFS.

The consensus from all the research on CFS and immune function is that the syndrome is characterized by a number of different immune system abnormalities which can vary from one patient to the next.

Immunologic Abnormalities Reported for CFS

Elevated levels of antibodies to viral proteins

Decreased natural killer cell activity

Low or elevated total antibody levels

Increased or decreased levels of circulating immune complexes

Increased cytokine (e.g., interleukin-2) levels

Decreased interferon levels

Altered helper/suppressor T-cell ratio

Fibromyalgia and CFS

Fibromyalgia, like CFS, is a recently recognized disorder regarded as a common cause of chronic musculoskeletal pain and fatigue. In fact, fibromyalgia and CFS may be one and the same.[3,4,11] The only difference in diagnostic criteria is the requirement of musculoskeletal pain in fibromyalgia and fatigue in CFS. The likelihood of being diagnosed with either is dependent upon the type of physician you consult. Specifically, if you are seeing a rheumatologist or orthopedic specialist, you are much more likely to be diagnosed with fibromyalgia.

Diagnostic Criteria for Fibromyalgia

Diagnosis requires fulfillment of all three major criteria and four or more minor criteria.

Major Criteria

Generalized aches or stiffness of at least three anatomic sites for at least three months

Six or more typical, reproducible tender points

Exclusion of other disorders which can cause similar symptoms

Minor Criteria

Generalized fatigue

Chronic headache

Sleep disturbance

Neurological and psychological complaints

Joint swelling

Numbing or tingling sensations

Irritable bowel syndrome

Variation of symptoms depending on activity, stress, and weather changes

Chapter Summary

Much attention has been focused lately on chronic fatigue syndrome. Although a newly defined illness, its symptoms have been around a long time. CFS can be a debilitating illness characterized by severe persistent fatigue along with other symptoms including low-grade fever, frequent sore throat, joint and muscle pain, and various neuro/psychological symptoms including depression.

Central to CFS is a disturbed immune system. While research has focused on trying to identify a specific infectious organism, CFS is more likely due to a general immune system failure.

Effective treatment of CFS must be comprehensive and address underlying factors which contribute to the weakened status of the immune system.

2

Diagnosing the Causes of Chronic Fatigue

This chapter will take you through the diagnostic process that I follow in my clinical practice when I am faced with the complaint of chronic fatigue. To effectively overcome chronic fatigue, even in the case of confirmed CFS, it is extremely important that as many contributing factors be identified as possible. In most instances I find more than one factor responsible for the symptom of fatigue.

The Medical Definition of Chronic Fatigue

Chronic fatigue is defined by doctors in several ways, including:

1. A state of abnormal exhaustion following normal activities
2. Decreased energy for tasks requiring sustained effort or attention

3. An overall inability to function effectively due to lack of energy

What Can Cause Chronic Fatigue?

A variety of physical and psychological factors contributing to chronic fatigue are listed below. The order is representative of how common the cause is among sufferers in the general population, based on the findings of several large studies as well as my clinical experience. Chronic fatigue syndrome is not the same as chronic fatigue and appears in this list under a broader category, impaired immune function.

Causes of Chronic Fatigue
Pre-existing Physical Condition
    Diabetes
    Heart disease
    Lung disease
    Rheumatoid arthritis
    Chronic inflammation
    Chronic pain
    Cancer
    Liver disease
    Multiple sclerosis
Prescription Drugs
    Anti-hypertensives
    Anti-inflammatory agents
    Birth control pills
    Antihistamines
    Corticosteroids
    Tranquilizers and sedatives

Depression

Stress/Low adrenal function

Impaired liver function and/or environmental illness

Impaired immune function

    Chronic fatigue syndrome

    Chronic candida infection

    Other chronic infections

Food allergies

Hypothyroidism

Hypoglycemia

Anemia and nutritional deficiencies

Sleep disturbance

Unknown cause

Clinical Evaluation of Chronic Fatigue

Many factors are considered when evaluating a patient with chronic fatigue. So how do I go about identifying the most important cause of a patient's fatigue? I start with a comprehensive patient questionnaire which includes the patient's medical history along with a series of questions organized in categories of body function. The answers provide a detailed review of different body systems. Some sections from my questionnaire are contained in this chapter.

Before I examine a patient for the first time, I study the questionnaire to familiarize myself with the case and I formulate a series of questions to gain more information if needed. I then sit down with the patient and get to know them on a personal level before we focus on their medical condition. My goal is to identify any factors which may be contributing to the patient's feeling of fatigue. Sometimes this is easy. For example, if a patient has heart disease, diabetes, or some other health condition, the condition or the drug they are taking is often clearly responsible for their fatigue. Treatment of the fatigue will be secondary to the treatment of the underlying health condition.

Further evaluation is often needed. The next steps can include a complete physical exam and laboratory studies. During the physical exam, I look for any clues to the cause for the chronic fatigue. For example, swollen lymph nodes may indicate a chronic infection, and the presence of a diagonal crease on both ear lobes usually indicates impaired blood flow to the brain, a significant cause of fatigue in the elderly.

I avoid ordering expensive laboratory tests unless they are absolutely necessary. However, I will usually order a complete blood count (CBC) and chemistry panel. The patient cost for these tests is about $30. I have the laboratory freeze the serum in case any further tests are needed after I review the results, so the patient won't be subjected to another blood draw. The initial blood tests I recommend for patients with chronic fatigue, a complete blood count and chemistry panel, break down the information I will need for my evaluation.

Recommended Initial Blood Tests
in Chronic Fatigue Patients
Complete Blood Count (CBC)

WBC count	RDW
RBC count	Platelet count
RBC morphology	Differential
Hemoglobin	Neutrophils
MCV	Lymphocytes
MCH	Monocytes
MCHC	Eosinophils

Erythrocyte sedimentation rate

Chemistry Panel

  Sodium

  Potassium

  Chloride

  CO_2

  Anion Gap

  Protein

  Albumin

  Globulin

  A/G ratio

  LDH

  AST (SGOT)

  ALT (SGPT)

  Bilirubin

    Total

    Direct

Alkaline phosphatase

Calcium

Phosphorus

Uric acid

BUN/Creatinine

Glucose

Cholesterol

Triglycerides

Thyroid panel

  T_3 uptake

  Thyroxine

  Free thyroxine index

Ferritin (women only)

I may order additional tests after the patient interview and studying the questionnaire. The following conditions should be ruled out before spending a lot of money on unnecessary lab studies:

Depression

Stress and low adrenal function

Impaired liver function and/or environmental illness

Impaired immune function and/or chronic infection

Food allergies

Hypothyroidism

Hypoglycemia

The methods I use for ruling out these conditions follow. Laboratory tests to confirm a diagnosis that is not going to effect treatment are unnecessary. For example, if it is quite obvious that an individual has an impaired immunity, it doesn't make much sense to perform elaborate and expensive blood tests on immune function, because the results of these tests are not likely to influence the method of treatment.

Depression

In the absence of a pre-existing physical condition, such as those described previously, depression is thought to be the most common cause of chronic fatigue. However, it is often difficult to determine whether the depression preceded the fatigue or vice versa.

Nearly one in four individuals will experience clinical depression in their lifetime. Clinical depression can be diagnosed via a number of different interview techniques and patient questionnaires. Here is a list of symptoms commonly associated with depression.

1. Poor appetite with weight loss, or increased appetite with weight gain
2. Insomnia or hypersomnia
3. Hyperactivity or inactivity
4. Loss of interest or pleasure in usual activities, or decrease in sex drive
5. Lack of energy or feelings of fatigue
6. Feelings of low self-esteem or inappropriate guilt
7. Diminished ability to think or concentrate
8. Recurrent thoughts of death or suicide

The presence of 5 of the 8 symptoms definitely indicates depression; the presence of 4 indicates probable depression.

Dealing with Depression

Depression can be caused by many of the same factors which cause chronic fatigue, and the natural approach to treating depression is similar to the natural approach to chronic fatigue. In addition to organic factors like food allergies, hypoglycemia, and nutrient deficiency, social and psychological factors can be underlying causes of depression. Chapter 3 discusses depression in more detail, including guidelines to help tune up the mind and attitude. If additional support is needed I might recommend the herb St. John's wort (see Chapter 11).

Stress and Low Adrenal Function

Stress can be an underlying factor in the patient with depression, low immune function, or chronic fatigue. To determine the role that stress may play, I rely a lot on my clinical judgment. I also utilize a popular method of rating stress levels, the Social Readjustment Rating Scale developed by Holmes and Rahe (Table 2.1).[1] The scale was originally designed to predict the likelihood of a person getting a serious disease due to stress. Various life-change events are numerically rated according to their potential for causing disease. Notice that even positive events, such as an outstanding personal achievement, can induce stress.

Interpreting Your Score

The standard interpretation of the Social Readjustment Rating scale is that a total of 200 or more units in one year increases the likelihood of getting a serious disease. I also utilize the scale to gain insight into a person's individual stress level. Not everyone reacts to stressful events in the same way. If it appears that a person has endured a fair amount of stress over a few months or longer, I will take measures to support the adrenal glands (see Chapter 9).

Table 2.1   Social Readjustment Rating Scale

Rank	Life Event	Mean Value
1	Death of spouse	100
2	Divorce	73
3	Marital separation	65
4	Jail term	63
5	Death of a close family member	63
6	Personal injury or illness	53
7	Marriage	50
8	Fired at work	47
9	Marital reconciliation	45
10	Retirement	45
11	Change in health of family member	44
12	Pregnancy	40
13	Sex difficulties	39
14	Gain of a new family member	39
15	Business adjustment	39
16	Change in financial state	38
17	Death of a close friend	37
18	Change to different line of work	36
19	Change in number of arguments with spouse	35
20	Large mortgage	31
21	Foreclosure of mortgage or loan	30
22	Change in responsibilities at work	29
23	Son or daughter leaving home	29
24	Trouble with in-laws	29
25	Outstanding personal achievement	28
26	Wife begins or stops work	26
27	Begin or end school	26
28	Change in living conditions	25
29	Revision of personal habits	24
30	Trouble with boss	23
31	Change in work hours or conditions	20
32	Change in residence	20
33	Change in schools	20
34	Change in recreation	19

Table 2.1   *(continued)*

Rank	Life Event	Mean Value
35	Change in church activities	19
36	Change in social activities	18
37	Small mortgage	17
38	Change in sleeping habits	16
39	Change in number of family get-togethers	15
40	Change in eating habits	15
41	Vacation	13
42	Christmas	12
43	Minor violations of the law	11

Dealing with Stress and Low Adrenal Function

Learning to deal effectively with stress involves both psychological and physiological support. Psychological relief can come from using the techniques in Chapter 3. Physiological support is comprehensively addressed in Chapters 5 and 9.

If you think that stress may be playing a major role in your feelings of fatigue, I encourage you to read the Getting Well Naturally title *Stress, Anxiety, and Insomnia.*

Impaired Liver Function and/or Environmental Illness

We all live in a polluted environment. Toxic substances are everywhere, in the air we breathe, the food we eat, and the water we drink. Even our bodies and the bacteria in the intestines produce toxic substances. Now more than ever, your health, the health of your immune system, and your energy levels are critically tied to your liver's ability to "detoxify."

Exposure or toxicity to food additives, solvents such as cleaning products, formaldehyde, toluene, and benzene, pesticides, herbicides, heavy metals (lead, mercury, cadmium, arsenic, nickel, and aluminum), and other toxic chemicals can greatly stress the liver's detoxification processes. This exposure can lead to a condition labeled by many naturopathic and nutrition-oriented physicians as the "congested liver" or "sluggish liver." These terms signify a reduced ability of the liver to detoxify. The congested or sluggish liver is characterized by a diminished bile flow, a condition known in medical terms as cholestasis. Besides exposure to toxic chemicals, impairment of bile flow within the liver can be caused by a variety of other agents and conditions, as listed below.

Causes of Cholestasis
Dietary factors
    Saturated fat
    Refined sugar
    Low fiber intake
Obesity
Diabetes
Gallstones
Alcohol
Endotoxins and other gut-derived bacterial toxins
Hereditary disorders such as Gilbert's syndrome
Pregnancy
Natural and synthetic steroid hormones
    Anabolic steroids
    Estrogen
    Oral contraceptives

Toxic chemicals or drugs
   Cleaning solvents
   Pesticides
   Antibiotics
   Diuretics
   Nonsteroidal anti-inflammatory drugs
   Thyroid hormone
Viral hepatitis

Although many of these conditions are typically associated with alterations in laboratory tests of liver function (serum bilirubin, AST, ALT, LDH, GGTP, etc.), relying on these tests alone to evaluate liver function may not be adequate, as these tests show elevation only when the liver has been significantly damaged. Many of these conditions in the initial or "subclinical" stages can show normal laboratory values.

Nutrition-oriented physicians will often use more sensitive tests to determine the functional activity of the liver, such as the serum bile acid assay and various clearance tests, but clinical judgment based on medical history remains the major diagnostic tool for the sluggish liver. The presence of chronic fatigue is the hallmark symptom.

Other symptoms that people with a sluggish liver may complain of are depression, general malaise, headache, digestive disturbance, allergies and chemical sensitivities, premenstrual syndrome, and constipation. Not surprisingly, these are the same symptoms experienced by people exposed to toxic chemicals. Many toxic chemicals (especially solvents) and heavy metals can affect nervous tissue, giving rise to a variety of psychological and neurological symptoms: depression, headache, mental confusion, mental illness, tingling in the extremities, abnormal nerve reflexes, and other signs of impaired nervous system function.[2,3]

A hair mineral analysis is a good screening test for heavy metal toxicity. If the hair mineral analysis is inconclusive, a more sensitive indicator is the 8-hour lead mobilization test. This test employs the chelating agent EDTA (edetate calcium disodium) and measures the level of lead excreted in the urine for a period of 8 hours after the injection of EDTA. The lead mobilization test must be performed by a licensed physician.

In the United States, the typical person has more lead and other heavy metals in their body than is compatible with good health. It is conservatively estimated that up to 25% of the United States population suffers from heavy metal poisoning to some extent.[3] The lead comes primarily from industrial sources and leaded gasoline. Each year more than 600,000 tons of lead is being dumped into our atmosphere and then inhaled or ingested. Other common sources of heavy metal poisoning are lead from the solder in tin cans, pesticide sprays, and cooking utensils; cadmium and lead from cigarette smoke; mercury from dental fillings, contaminated fish, and cosmetics; and aluminum from antacids and cookware. Some professions with extremely high exposure include battery makers, gas station attendants, printers, roofers, solderers, dentists, and jewelers.

Enhancing Liver Function and Detoxification

Aiding the liver and detoxification involves: (1) adopting a healthy lifestyle including regular exercise; (2) eating a diet of fresh fruits and vegetables, whole grains, legumes, nuts, and seeds; (3) taking a high-potency multiple vitamin and mineral supplement; (4) using special nutritional and herbal supplements to enhance liver function; and (5) going on a 3-day fast at the change of each season.

See Chapter 7 for more information on chronic fatigue and liver function.

Impaired Immune Function and/or Chronic Infection

The role that an impaired immune system plays in chronic fatigue syndrome was discussed in Chapter 1. When the immune system is impaired, infections can linger and fatigue can persist. There is a good reason for fatigue during an infection—your immune system works best when the body is at rest.

To determine the extent that the immune system is implicated in patients with chronic fatigue, I employ a series of questions. An answer of yes to any of the following questions usually indicates that the immune system needs support.

- Do you get more than 2 colds per year?
- When you catch a cold, does it take more than 5 to 7 days to get rid of the symptoms?
- Have you ever had infectious mononucleosis?
- Do you have herpes?
- Do you suffer from chronic infections of any kind?

Chronic Candida Infection

One of the most frequent findings in individuals with low immune function is an overgrowth of the common yeast Candida albicans. Normally, candida lives harmlessly in the gastrointestinal tract. However, sometimes candida will overgrow, leading indirectly to significant disease or directly invading body tissues.

Factors Predisposing Individuals to Candida Overgrowth
Impaired immune function
Anti-ulcer drugs
Broad-spectrum antibiotics

Cellular immunodeficiency
Corticosteroids
Diabetes mellitus
Excessive sugar in the diet
Intravascular catheters
Intravenous drug use
Lack of digestive secretions
Oral contraceptive agents

Candidal overgrowth is now recognized as a complex medical syndrome known as the yeast syndrome or chronic candidiasis. This overgrowth is believed to cause a wide variety of symptoms in virtually every system of the body, with the gastrointestinal, genitourinary, endocrine, nervous, and immune systems being the most susceptible. Figure 2.1 shows the typical chronic candidiasis patient's profile.

Diagnosing Chronic Candidiasis

The diagnosis of chronic candidiasis is often quite difficult as there is no single specific diagnostic test. Stool cultures and elevated antibody levels to candida are useful diagnostic aids, but they should not be exclusively relied upon. The best method is a detailed medical history and patient questionnaire. Figure 2.2, shown on page 28, shows the questionnaire that I use.

Dealing with Chronic Candidiasis

Seven important steps to successfully control Candida albicans are outlined as follows.

1. Eliminate the use of antibiotics, steroids, immune-suppressing drugs, and birth control pills (unless there is absolute medical necessity).

Sex: Female

Age: 15–50

General symptoms:
　Chronic fatigue
　Lack of energy
　General malaise
　Decreased libido

Gastrointestinal symptoms:
　Thrush
　Bloating, gas
　Intestinal cramps
　Rectal itching
　Altered bowel function

Genitourinary system complaints:
　Vaginal yeast infection
　Frequent bladder infections

Endocrine system complaints:
　Primarily menstrual complaints

Nervous system complaints:
　Depression
　Irritability
　Inability to concentrate

Immune system complaints:
　Allergies
　Chemical sensitivities
　Low immune function

Past history:
　Chronic vaginal yeast infections
　Chronic antibiotic use for infections or acne
　Oral birth control usage
　Oral steroid hormone usage

Associated conditions:
　Premenstrual syndrome
　Sensitivity to foods, chemicals, and other allergens
　Endocrine disturbances
　Psoriasis
　Irritable bowel syndrome

Other:
　Craving for foods rich in carbohydrates or yeast

Figure 2.1　Typical chronic candidiasis patient profile

History	Point Score
1. Have you taken antibiotics for acne for one month or longer?	25
2. Have you, at any time in your life, taken other "broad spectrum" antibiotics for respiratory, urinary, or other infections for two months or longer, or in short courses four or more times in a one-year period?	20
3. Have you ever taken a broad spectrum antibiotic— even a single course?	6
4. Have you, at any time in your life, been bothered by persistent prostatitis, vaginitis, or other problems affecting your reproductive organs?	25
5. Have you been pregnant . . .	
One time?	3
Two or more times?	5
6. Have you taken birth control pills . . .	
For six months to two years?	8
For more than two years?	15
7. Have you taken prednisone or other cortisone-type drugs . . .	
For two weeks or less?	6
For more than two weeks?	15
8. Does exposure to perfumes, insecticides, fabric shop odors, and other chemicals provoke . . .	
Mild symptoms?	5
Moderate to severe symptoms?	20
9. Are your symptoms worse on damp, muggy days or in moldy places?	20
10. Have you had athlete's foot, ringworm, "jock itch," or other chronic infections of the skin or nails?	
Mild to moderate?	10
Severe or persistent?	20
11. Do you crave sugar?	10
12. Do you crave breads?	10
13. Do you crave alcoholic beverages?	10
14. Does tobacco smoke *really* bother you?	10
Total Score	▬▬▬

Figure 2.2   The candida questionnaire

Major Symptoms

For each of your symptoms, enter the appropriate figure
in the Point Score column.

If a symptom is occasional or mild score 3 points.

If a symptom is frequent and/or moderately severe score 6 points.

If a symptom is severe and/or disabling score 9 points.

Point Score

1. Fatigue or lethargy _____
2. Feeling of being "drained" _____
3. Poor memory _____
4. Feeling "spacey" or "unreal" _____
5. Depression _____
6. Numbness, burning, or tingling _____
7. Muscle aches _____
8. Muscle weakness or paralysis _____
9. Pain and/or swelling in joints _____
10. Abdominal pain _____
11. Constipation _____
12. Diarrhea _____
13. Bloating _____
14. Persistent vaginal itch _____
15. Persistent vaginal burning _____
16. Prostatitis _____
17. Impotence _____
18. Loss of sexual desire _____
19. Endometriosis _____
20. Cramps and/or other menstrual irregularities _____
21. Premenstrual tension _____
22. Spots in front of eyes _____
23. Erratic vision _____

Total Score ▬▬▬

Figure 2.2   *(continued)*

Other Symptoms

For each of your symptoms, enter the appropriate figure
in the Point Score column.

If a symptom is occasional or mild score 1 point.

If a symptom is frequent and/or moderately severe score 2 points.

If a symptom is severe and/or disabling score 3 points.

Point Score

1. Drowsiness   _____
2. Irritability   _____
3. Incoordination   _____
4. Inability to concentrate   _____
5. Frequent mood swings   _____
6. Headache   _____
7. Dizziness/loss of balance   _____
8. Pressure above ears, feeling of head swelling and tingling   _____
9. Itching   _____
10. Other rashes   _____
11. Heartburn   _____
12. Indigestion   _____
13. Belching and intestinal gas   _____
14. Mucus in stools   _____
15. Hemorrhoids   _____
16. Dry mouth   _____
17. Rash or blisters in mouth   _____
18. Bad breath   _____
19. Joint swelling or arthritis   _____
20. Nasal congestion or discharge   _____
21. Postnasal drip   _____
22. Nasal itching   _____
23. Sore or dry throat   _____
24. Cough   _____
25. Pain or tightness in chest   _____
26. Wheezing or shortness of breath   _____

Figure 2.2   *(continued)*

	Point Score
27. Urinary urgency or frequency	———
28. Burning on urination	———
29. Failing vision	———
30. Burning or tearing of eyes	———
31. Recurrent infections or fluid in ears	———
32. Ear pain or deafness	———

Total Score ━━━━━━━

Total Score of All Three Sections ━━━━━━━

Interpretation	Women	Men
Yeast-connected health problems are almost certainly present	>180	>140
Yeast-connected health problems are probably present	120–180	90–140
Yeast-connected health problems are possibly present	60–119	40–89
Yeast-connected health problems are less likely present	<60	<40

Adapted from Crook WG: *The Yeast Connection,* 2nd ed. Professional Books, Jackson, TN, 1984

Figure 2.2   *(continued)*

2. Follow special dietary guidelines (see also Chapter 4):
   Avoid foods high in simple carbohydrate content such as refined sugars (sucrose, fructose, corn syrup), processed fruit juices, honey, and maple syrup.

   Avoid foods with a high content of yeast or mold including alcoholic beverages, cheeses, dried fruits, melons, and peanuts. These foods promote candida overgrowth.

Avoid milk and milk products due to their high content of lactose (milk sugar) and trace levels of antibiotics. Avoid all known or suspected allergens since allergies can weaken the immune system and provide a more hospitable environment for the yeast.

3. Enhance digestive function with the use of hydrochloric acid and/or pancreatic enzymes.

4. Enhance liver function (see Chapter 7).

5. Enhance immune function (see Chapter 8).

6. Use nutritional and herbal supplements which help control against yeast overgrowth and promote a healthy bacterial flora.

7. Eliminate candida toxins by using a water-soluble fiber source such as guar gum, psyllium seed, or pectin which can bind to toxins in the gut and promote their excretion.

Food Allergies

As far back as 1930, noted allergist Dr. Albert Rowe began noticing that chronic fatigue was a key feature of food allergies.[3] Originally, Dr. Rowe described a syndrome known as "allergic toxemia" to describe a syndrome that included the symptoms of fatigue, muscle and joint aches, drowsiness, poor concentration, nervousness, and depression. During the 1950s, this syndrome began to be referred to as the allergic tension-fatigue syndrome.[4] With the current prevalence of CFS as a catch-all diagnosis many physicians and other people are forgetting that food allergies can lead to chronic fatigue. Furthermore, between 55% and 85% of individuals with CFS are found to have food allergies.

A food allergy occurs when there is an adverse reaction to the ingestion of a food. The reaction may or may not be mediated by the immune system. A bad reaction may be caused by a food protein, starch, or other food component, or by contaminants in the food such as colorings or preservatives. Other terms often used for food allergy include: food hypersensitivity, food anaphylaxis, food idiosyncrasy, food intolerance, pharmacological (drug-like) reaction to food, metabolic reaction to food, and food sensitivity. The number of people suffering from food allergies has increased dramatically during the last 15 years. Some physicians believe that food allergies are the leading cause of most undiagnosed symptoms and that at least 60% of the American population suffers from symptoms associated with food reactions.[5] Theories of why the incidence has increased include: increased stresses on the immune system (such as greater chemical pollution in our air, water, and food), earlier weaning and earlier introduction of solid foods to infants, genetic manipulation of plants resulting in food components with greater allergenic tendencies, and increased ingestion of fewer foods. Probably all of these and more have contributed to the increased frequency and severity of symptoms.

Two basic categories of tests are commonly used to diagnose food allergies: (1) food challenge and (2) laboratory methods. Each has its advantages. Food challenge methods add no additional expense, but require a great deal of individual motivation. Laboratory procedures such as blood tests can provide immediate identification of suspected allergens, but they can be expensive.

Food Challenge Test for Food Allergies

Many physicians believe that oral food challenge is the best way of diagnosing food sensitivities. There are two broad categories of food challenge testing: (1) elimination (also known as oligoantigenic) diet, followed by food reintroduction, and (2) pure water fast, followed by food challenge. *A note of caution: food challenge testing should NOT be used in people with symptoms that are potentially life threatening (such as airway constriction or severe allergic reactions).*

In the elimination diet method you are placed on a limited diet; commonly eaten foods are eliminated and replaced with either hypoallergenic foods and foods rarely eaten, or special hypoallergenic formulas. The fewer the allergic foods the greater the ease of establishing a diagnosis with an elimination diet. The standard elimination diet consists of lamb, chicken, potatoes, rice, banana, apple, and a cabbage family vegetable (cabbage, Brussels sprouts, broccoli, etc.). Variations of the elimination diet are possible, however, it is extremely important that no allergic foods be consumed.

The individual stays on this limited diet for at least one week, up to one month. If the symptoms are related to food sensitivity, they will typically disappear by the fifth or sixth day of the diet. If the symptoms do not disappear, it is possible that a food in the elimination diet is responsible, in which case an even more restricted diet must be utilized.

After one week, individual foods are reintroduced every two days. Methods range from reintroducing only a single food every two days, to one every one or two meals. Usually after the one-week "cleansing" period, the patient will develop a noticeable, increased sensitivity to the offending foods, a more severe or recognizable symptom than before. A careful, detailed record must be maintained describing which foods were reintroduced and when, and what symptoms appeared. It can be very useful to track the wrist pulse during reintroduction, as pulse changes may occur when an allergic food is consumed.

For many people, elimination diets offer the most viable means of detection of a food allergy. Because one can dramatically experience the effects of food reactions, motivation to eliminate the offending food can be high. The only down side of this procedure is that it is time-consuming and requires discipline and motivation.

Laboratory Methods to Diagnose Food Allergies

The skin prick or skin scratch test employed by many allergists only tests for allergies mediated by a particular antibody known as IgE. As only 10% to 15% of all food allergies are mediated by IgE, this test is of little value in diagnosing most food allergies. In the skin prick test, food extracts are placed on the patient's skin with a scratch or prick method. If the patient is allergic to the food, a welt will form immediately as the allergen reacts with IgE-sensitized cells in the patient's skin.

A better route to follow in the laboratory diagnosis of food allergies is the use of special blood tests. The blood tests are extremely convenient and relatively accurate, but they tend to be expensive (around $200 for a full panel). The RAST (radio-allergo-sorbent test) and the ELISA (enzyme-linked immunosorbent assay) tests appear to be the best laboratory methods currently available.

Dealing with Food Allergies

While there is no known simple "cure" for food allergies, some measures can be taken to help alleviate symptoms and correct the underlying causes. These measures are detailed in Chapter 4.

Hypothyroidism

Hypothyroidism (low thyroid function), a common cause of chronic fatigue, is often overlooked by many physicians. The reason may be their reliance on blood measurements of thyroid hormone levels for diagnosis.

Before physicians began using blood tests for thyroid hormone levels, it was common to diagnose hypothyroidism based on basal body temperature (the temperature of the body at rest) and Achilles reflex time (reflexes are slowed in hypothyroidism). Many physicians still claim that these "functional" tests are more sensitive in diagnosing hypothyroidism than standard blood tests. This opinion holds particularly true in the diagnosis of milder forms of hypothyroidism. As mild hypothyroidism is more common, the majority of people with hypothyroidism are going undiagnosed.[6–8]

Undiagnosed hypothyroidism is a serious concern, as failure to treat this as an underlying condition reduces the effectiveness of every other measure designed to increase energy levels. It is like trying to run your car without a fuel pump. There may be plenty of gas in the tank, but it is not being delivered to the engine.

In my clinical practice, when I suspect hypothyroidism, I'll have the patient take their basal body temperature, as this is the most sensitive functional test of thyroid function.[6,7]

Taking Your Basal Body Temperature

Your body temperature reflects your metabolic rate, which is largely determined by hormones secreted by the thyroid gland. The function of the thyroid gland can be determined by simply measuring your basal body temperature. All you need is a thermometer.

Procedure

1. Shake down the thermometer to below 95°F and place it by your bed before going to sleep at night.
2. On waking, place the thermometer in your armpit for a full 10 minutes. It is important to make as little movement as possible. Lying and resting with your eyes closed is best. Do not get up until the 10-minute test is completed.

3. After 10 minutes, read and record the temperature and date.

4. Record your basal body temperature for at least three mornings (preferably at the same time of day). Menstruating women must perform the test on the second, third, and fourth days of menstruation. Men and post-menopausal women can perform the test at any time.

Interpretation Your basal body temperature should be between 97.6° and 98.2°. Low basal body temperatures are quite common and may reflect hypothyroidism. In addition to fatigue, common signs and symptoms of hypothyroidism are low basal body temperature, depression, difficulty in losing weight, dry skin, headache, menstrual problems, recurrent infections, constipation, and sensitivity to cold.

High basal body temperatures (above 98.6°) are less common, but may be evidence of *hyper*thyroidism. Common signs and symptoms of hyperthyroidism include bulging eyeballs, fast pulse, hyperactivity, inability to gain weight, insomnia, irritability, menstrual problems, and nervousness.

Treatment of Hypothyroidism

The treatment of hypothyroidism is detailed in Chapter 10.

Hypoglycemia

Hypoglycemia (low blood sugar), another common cause of chronic fatigue, results from faulty carbohydrate (sugar) metabolism. The body strives to maintain blood sugar (glucose) levels within a narrow range primarily to assure the brain a constant and even supply of glucose, the brain's primary source of energy. Typically, symptoms of hypoglycemia affect the brain first.

Symptoms of hypoglycemia can range from mild to severe and include such things as: fatigue; headache; depression, anxiety, irritability, and other psychological disturbances; blurred vision; excessive sweating; mental confusion; incoherent speech; bizarre behavior; and convulsions. The association between hypoglycemia and fatigue is well-known. What is not as well-known is the part that hypoglycemia plays in contributing to depression. Numerous studies have shown that depressed individuals often suffer from hypoglycemia as well. Since depression is the most common cause of chronic fatigue, hypoglycemia must always be ruled out.

Diagnosing Hypoglycemia

The standard method of diagnosing hypoglycemia is the oral glucose tolerance test (GTT). It is used in the diagnosis of both hypoglycemia and diabetes, although it is rarely required for the latter. After fasting for at least 12 hours, a baseline blood glucose measurement is made. Then the subject is given a very sweet liquid containing glucose to drink. Blood sugar levels are re-checked at 30 minutes, 1 hour, and then hourly for up to 6 hours. Basically, if blood sugar levels rise to a level greater than 200 milligrams per deciliter it indicates diabetes. If levels fall below 50 milligrams per deciliter, it indicates reactive hypoglycemia. Hypoglycemia can also be diagnosed if there is a decrease of 20 milligrams or more from the fasting level after 4 hours. A diagnosis of probable reactive hypoglycemia is made if there is a decrease of 10 to 20 milligrams from the fasting level after 4 hours.

The Glucose-Insulin Tolerance Test

In diagnosing hypoglycemia, relying on blood sugar levels alone is often not enough. It is now widely recognized that signs and symptoms of hypoglycemia can occur in individuals having blood glucose levels well above 50 milligrams per deciliter.[9] Many of the symptoms linked to hypoglycemia appear to be a result of increases in insulin or epinephrine; therefore, it has been recommended that insulin or epinephrine (adrenaline) be measured at the same time. Symptoms often correlate better with elevations in these hormones than with glucose levels.[10,11] Several studies have shown that the glucose-insulin tolerance test (G-ITT) leads to a greater sensitivity in the diagnosis of hypoglycemia than the standard GTT.[11,12] As many as two-thirds of subjects with suspected diabetes or hypoglycemia who have normal glucose tolerance tests will demonstrate abnormal insulin tolerance tests. The down side to this test is that it tends to be very costly. For example, the glucose-insulin tolerance test (G-ITT) costs around $200 while a standard GTT is usually less than $30.

The Hypoglycemia Questionnaire

When all is considered (especially cost), the most useful measure of diagnosing hypoglycemia in many cases remains assessing symptoms. The hypoglycemia questionnaire (Figure 2.3) is an excellent screening method.

Treating Hypoglycemia

Following the dietary recommendations in Chapter 4 is usually all that is needed to re-establish proper control of blood sugar levels. In addition, taking supplemental chromium, as either chromium polynicotinate or chromium picolinate, can be very useful. Chromium is critical to proper blood sugar control.[13]

What If There Are Multiple Causes?

It is more likely that there are multiple causes for an individual's symptoms than no identifiable causes. Chapter 12

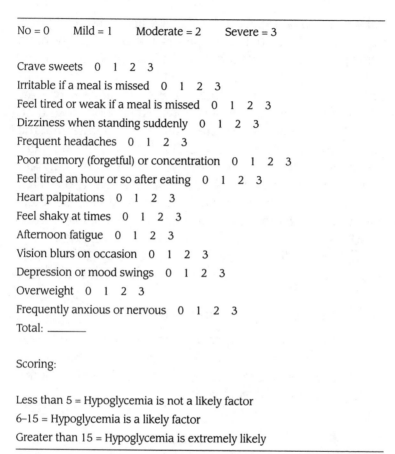

No = 0   Mild = 1   Moderate = 2   Severe = 3

Crave sweets   0   1   2   3
Irritable if a meal is missed   0   1   2   3
Feel tired or weak if a meal is missed   0   1   2   3
Dizziness when standing suddenly   0   1   2   3
Frequent headaches   0   1   2   3
Poor memory (forgetful) or concentration   0   1   2   3
Feel tired an hour or so after eating   0   1   2   3
Heart palpitations   0   1   2   3
Feel shaky at times   0   1   2   3
Afternoon fatigue   0   1   2   3
Vision blurs on occasion   0   1   2   3
Depression or mood swings   0   1   2   3
Overweight   0   1   2   3
Frequently anxious or nervous   0   1   2   3
Total: _____

Scoring:

Less than 5 = Hypoglycemia is not a likely factor
6–15 = Hypoglycemia is a likely factor
Greater than 15 = Hypoglycemia is extremely likely

Figure 2.3   The hypoglycemia questionnaire

provides guidelines to assess a priority to the various possible reasons for chronic fatigue. Fortunately, it is not difficult to work on many of the most obvious causes simultaneously as they tend to overlap.

Chapter Summary

Many factors can bring on the symptom of chronic fatigue. Successful treatment largely depends upon addressing the cause, so every effort should be made to identify all responsible factors. These can be identified via proper clinical evaluation by a physician along with some detective work by the patient. The comprehensive evaluation of chronic fatigue includes a detailed medical history, a thorough review of body systems (either by interview or questionnaire), and appropriate laboratory evaluation. Once the causes underlying the chronic fatigue are identified, an effective treatment plan can be implemented.

II

Foundational Approach to Chronic Fatigue

3

Tuning Up the Mind and Attitude

The ability of the mind to affect the process of virtually every disease has been well documented, and the internal mechanisms and pathways by which the mind can positively or negatively affect healing processes and the immune system have received considerable attention in the scientific literature.[1,2] As the body of knowledge confirmng the critical role of the psyche on health has grown, it has become quite clear that what we think and how we feel has a tremendous effect on the way our body functions.

Influence of the Mind on the Immune System

Psychoneuroimmunology is a scientific field which studies the influence that the mind and emotions have on immune function.[2] Although much still remains to be learned, what is known currently is that thoughts and emotions can indeed significantly impact the immune system. Basically, negative emotional states like depression, anger, fear, and grief have been shown to have a negative effect. Conversely, positive emotional states like love, joy, and laughter exert a positive effect on the immune system.[2,3]

Emotional State and Immune Function

It has been well accepted that negative emotional states adversely affect the immune system, but for some reason the medical community has scoffed at the notion that positive emotional states can enhance immune function.

Although it does not have to be a major life event to cause depressed immune function, it is safe to say that the more significant the stressor the greater the impact on the immune system. The loss of a spouse, a very stressful life event, was strongly associated with increased morbidity and mortality long before a link between the mind and immune function was documented. In fact, it was not until 1977 that a study of 26 bereaved spouses observed conclusively that grief led to a significant depression in immune function (natural killer cell activity was significantly reduced).[4] Subsequent studies have further demonstrated that bereavement, depression, and stress significantly diminish important immune functions.[2,3,5]

By the end of the 1970s, several studies had shown that negative emotions suppress immune function. In 1979, Norman Cousins' popular book *Anatomy of an Illness* caused a significant stir in the medical community. An autobiographical anecdotal account, the book postulated that positive emotional states can cure the body of even a quite serious disease.[6] Cousins watched *Candid Camera,* Marx brothers films, and read humorous books, and claimed that this was the cure.

At first, physicians and researchers scoffed at Cousins' concept. Now, however, it is being proven in numerous studies that laughter and other positive emotional states can in fact enhance the function of the immune system.[7,8] The use of guided imagery, hypnosis, and other meditative states have been shown to do the same.[2,3]

Emotional State and Chronic Fatigue

The link between CFS, emotional state, and immune function is clear. As detailed in Chapter 1, CFS is generally characterized by impaired immune function. The most consistent finding is low natural killer cell activity. Emotional states such as depression (or even boredom) are also characterized by impaired immunity, with one of the most consistent findings being low natural killer cell activity.[9,10]

Obviously, a good prescription if you suffer from CFS, or just chronic fatigue, is to watch comedies and laugh as much as possible. In addition, you can learn to program your mind and attitude for higher energy levels.

Programming Your Emotional State   Our emotional state plays a major role in determining our energy levels as well as the status of our immune system. When we are experiencing depression, grief, or sadness our energy levels will tend to be depressed. Conversely, if we are happy, joyful, and up our energy level goes up.

Many of the patients that I have seen with chronic fatigue or CFS are either depressed or just seem to have lost a sense of real enthusiasm for life. I realize that it's not easy to be enthusiastic if you do not have energy. But the two usually go hand in hand. Have you ever been dead tired, but all of a sudden found something to excite you to a point where you felt revitalized?

How energetic you feel at any given time depends upon a combination of two very simple factors: what your mind is focusing on and your physiology. Many people with chronic fatigue focus only on how tired they are. They say it over and over again, to themselves and to anyone else who will listen. Their physiology includes not only the chemicals and hormones floating around in the body, but also the way they hold their body (slouched posture) and how they breathe (shallowly). In most patients with chronic fatigue, both the mind and the body need tuning. This chapter focuses on the mind; the remaining chapters address changing the body's physiology.

As simple as the following recommendation is going to sound, believe me, it is effective. The first step on the way to having an abundance of energy is *believing that you can have an abundance of energy.* This step may be the most important one that you take. If you could imagine yourself having unlimited energy, what would it feel like? How would you be breathing? What would your body feel like? If you can imagine how it feels to have abundant energy, you can have it.

Importance of a Positive Attitude

It is becoming increasingly clear that the most important factor in maintaining or attaining health is a consistent "positive mental attitude." Researchers in the medical and psychological fields have demonstrated repeatedly that your level of optimism is a major factor in your level of wellness. Optimists view the misfortunes of life as temporary setbacks, challenges, or opportunities for growth. Research shows that optimists are healthier and may even live longer than pessimists.[11,12] I believe that optimists also have higher energy levels.

According to Martin Seligman, Ph.D., the world's leading authority on optimism, humans are by nature optimists, and optimism is a necessary step towards achieving our goals in life.[13] The first step in building an optimistic or positive mental attitude is to start taking personal responsibility for your own mental state, your life, your current situation, and your health. Then you can begin taking action to make the changes you desire.

Conditioning Your Mind and Attitude

Achieving and maintaining high self-esteem and a healthy, positive mental attitude are critical factors to health and high energy levels. You need to exercise or condition your attitude in much the same way you condition your body. I have developed some exercises to help you achieve the kind of permanent results you really want—by conditioning you for success.

First, you will need a notebook to write in, your personal journal. A journal is a powerful tool to help you stay in touch with your feelings, thoughts, and emotions. The exercises are the foundation to help you learn how to adopt healthier attitudes. Your daily personal journal will build upon this foundation.

Exercise #1   Creating a Positive Goal Statement

Learning to set goals that result in a positive experience is critical to your success. The following guidelines can be used to set any goal including your desired weight. Use successful goal setting to create a "success cycle." Achieving your goals helps you feel better about yourself. The better you feel about yourself, the more likely you will achieve your goals.

1. State the goal in positive terms; do not use any negative words. For example, it is better to say "I enjoy eating healthy, low-calorie, nutritious foods" than "I will not eat sugar, candy, ice cream, and other fattening foods."

2. Make your goal attainable and realistic. This creates a success cycle and new, positive self-image. Little things can add up to make a major difference in the way you feel about yourself.

3. Be specific. For example, say you want to have higher energy levels. What are some of the activities that you

want to enjoy? How exactly do you want to feel? Clearly define what it is you want to achieve, and you will be more likely to reach it.

4. State the goal in present tense, not future. See and feel yourself having already achieved the goal and what success feels like. As noted psychologist Dr. Wayne Dyer says "You'll see it, when you believe it." You must literally program yourself to achieve the goal.

Goal Statement   Use the guidelines in Exercise #1 to construct your own positive goal statement. Example: "My body is strong and full of energy. I am running two miles three times a week. I feel good about myself and my body. I am gaining more energy every day by focusing on how much energy I already have. I am making healthy food choices. I feel fantastic!!" Write your positive goal statement in your notebook.

Short-Term Goals

Any voyage begins with one step. Meeting your short-term goals will help you achieve the long-term results you described in your positive goal statement. Get in the habit of asking yourself each morning and evening: What must I do today to achieve my long-term goal?

Exercise #2   The Power of Questions

According to Anthony Robbins, author of the bestsellers *Unlimited Power* and *Awaken the Giant Within,* the quality of your life is equal to the quality of the questions you habitually ask yourself. This is based on the belief that whatever question you ask your brain, you will get an answer.

Consider the following example: An individual is met with a particular challenge or problem. He or she can now ask a number of questions: "Why does this always happen to me?" Or, "Why am I always so stupid?" Do they get answers to these questions? Do the answers build self-esteem? Does the problem keep reappearing? What would be a higher quality question? How about, "This is a very interesting situation, what do I need to learn from this so that it never happens again?" Or how about, "What can I do to make this situation better?"

Now let's look at an individual who suffers from chronic fatigue. What questions are they asking themselves which are not helping their situation? "Why am I always so tired? Why don't I have any energy? Why doesn't anything I try to increase my energy ever seem to work?"

Some better questions to ask yourself would be: "What do I need to do to gain more energy? How can I gain more energy and have fun at the same time? What do I need to commit to in order to have more energy?" After you have answered these questions, answer this one: "If I had high energy right now, what would it feel like?"

As the mind searches for answers to your questions, it is reprogramming your subconscious into believing that you have an abundance of energy. Unless there is a physiological reason for your chronic fatigue, it won't take long before your subconscious believes.

Regardless of your physical situation, asking better questions is bound to improve your attitude. If you want to have a better life, simply ask better questions. It sounds simple, because it is. To help you achieve more energy, excitement, and happiness in your life, use your personal journal to ask yourself the following questions on a consistent basis.

The Morning Questions

1. What am I most happy about in my life right now?
   Why does that make me happy?
   How does that make me feel?

2. What am I most excited about in my life right now?
   Why does that make me excited?
   How does that make me feel?
3. What am I most grateful for in my life right now?
   Why does that make me grateful?
   How does that make me feel?
4. What am I enjoying most about my life right now?
   What about that do I enjoy?
   How does that make me feel?
5. What am I committed to in my life right now?
   Why am I committed to that?
   How does that make me feel?
6. Who do I love? (Start close and move out.)
7. Who loves me?
8. What will I do today to achieve my long-term goal?

The Evening Questions
1. What have I given today?
   In what ways have I been a giver today?
2. What did I learn today?
3. What did I do today to reach my long-term goal?
4. In what ways was today a perfect day?
5. Repeat morning questions.

Problem or Challenge Questions
1. What is right/great about this problem that I am faced with?
2. What is not perfect yet?
3. What am I willing to do to make it the way I want?
4. How can I enjoy doing those things that are necessary to make it the way I want it?

Exercise #3 *Affirmations*

An affirmation is a statement. It can be either positive or negative. Affirmations can make imprints on the subconscious mind to create a healthy, positive self-image or they can be used to rot away at your self-esteem and confidence. An example of a positive affirmation on energy levels would be "I have an abundance of energy." A negative affirmation would be "I am exhausted."

Affirmations can fuel the changes you desire. Let me give you some guidelines for creating your own positive affirmations.

Always phrase your affirmation in the present tense.

Always phrase the affirmation in a positive way and totally associate to the positive feelings that are generated.

Keep the affirmation short and simple, but full of feeling. Be creative.

Imagine yourself really experiencing what you are affirming. The more you can identify with the affirmation, the more powerful it becomes.

Make the affirmation personal and full of meaning.

Here are some examples of positive affirmations.

1. I am a whole and complete person.
2. I am in control of my life.
3. I am an open channel of love and joy.
4. I am full of energy.
5. I am good to my body.
6. I am growing stronger every day.
7. I am energetic, excited, and enthusiastic.

Create Your Own Affirmations

Using my guidelines and examples, write down five affirmations that apply to you. State these affirmations out loud for five minutes every day. The more you can associate or attach your feelings to the affirmation, the stronger it imprints upon your subconscious mind. Choose a place that is comfortable and quiet, and a time when you will not be interrupted or disturbed. Sit or lie in a comfortable position. Begin by taking ten deep breaths: inhale to a count of one, hold for a count of two, exhale to a count of four. Now write down your positive affirmations. Read them out loud. Start believing in the power of a positive attitude.

Chapter Summary

As researchers have sought to understand the complex interrelationship between the mind and body, there is a growing awareness of the importance that attitude and emotional states play in determining health and disease. With increased understanding, we are learning to use techniques to enhance the immune system and other body functions by accessing the tremendous power of the human mind.

The techniques detailed in this chapter are designed to help increase your energy level, and build a foundation of healthy self-esteem and a positive attitude. Growth in these areas usually happens by degrees, subtle changes accumulating one by one. Would you be in good physical condition if you only exercised once? No way. It takes conditioning. You can, with practice, have a positive attitude and high self-esteem.

4

Dietary Guidelines

Your energy level is directly related to the quality of the foods you routinely ingest. The human body is the most remarkable machine in the world, but most Americans are not feeding it the high-quality fuel it deserves. When a machine does not receive proper fuel or maintenance, how long can it be expected to run in an efficient manner? If your body is not fed the full range of nutrients it needs, how can it be expected to stay in a state of good health?

Instead of eating foods rich in vital nutrients, most Americans live on refined foods high in calories, sugar, fat, and cholesterol. Instead of life-giving foods, Americans are filling up on cheeseburgers, french fries, Twinkies, and chocolate chip cookies, and washing them down with artificially colored and flavored fruit drinks or colas. It is an undeniable fact that the three leading causes of death in the United States (heart disease, cancer, and stroke) are diet-related and that over one-third of our adult population is overweight.

Dietary Guidelines for Chronic Fatigue

Individuals who suffer from chronic fatigue need supernutrition. They need high-quality foods for fuel and they need to avoid those foods which rob the body of energy. This chapter details the dietary guidelines that I recommend in the treatment of chronic fatigue.

Basic Guidelines

1. Eliminate or restrict your intake of caffeine.
2. Eliminate refined carbohydrates.
3. Buy and use a juicer.
4. Design a healthful diet.
5. Eat regular, planned meals.
6. Rotate foods to prevent food allergies.

Caffeine and Energy Levels

Caffeine-containing beverages and herbs—coffee, tea, guarana, cola nut, and cocoa—are used worldwide to help us fight off fatigue. Moderate consumption may be helpful in relieving fatigue temporarily in some cases, however, overconsumption can result in significant side effects, including "caffeinism," a medical condition characterized by symptoms of depression, nervousness, irritability, recurrent headache, heart palpitations, and insomnia.

The average American consumes 150 to 225 milligrams of caffeine each day, roughly the amount of caffeine in one to two cups of coffee. Although most people can handle this amount, some are more sensitive to the effects of caffeine due to a slower elimination from the body. Even small amounts of caffeine, as found in decaffeinated coffee, are enough to affect some people adversely and produce caffeinism.[1] Table 4.1 shows the relative caffeine content in our most popular beverages.

Caffeine in relatively small doses (50 to 200 milligrams) stimulates the brain areas associated with conscious mental processes. The result is your ideas become clearer, thoughts flow more easily and rapidly, and fatigue and drowsiness decrease. Typists, for example, work faster and with fewer errors after ingesting caffeine, and drivers will notice that caffeine can increase alertness and improve their driving performance.[1]

However, the anti-fatigue effects of caffeine are usually short-lived. After the initial simulation a period of increased fatigue often results. A vicious cycle can then ensue in which a person drinks increasing amounts of caffeine to delay the onset of fatigue.[2]

Long-term use of caffeine-containing beverages, especially coffee, should be avoided. There is evidence that *chronic caffeine intake may actually lead to chronic fatigue.* While mice fed one dose of caffeine demonstrated significant

Table 4.1   Caffeine Content of Coffee, Tea, and Selected Soft Drinks

Beverage	Caffeine Content (in milligrams)	Beverage	Caffeine Content (in milligrams)
Coffee (7.5-ounce cup)		*Soft drinks*	
Drip	115+	Jolt	100
Brewed	80–135	Mountain Dew	54
Instant	65–40	Tab	47
Decaffeinated	3–4	Coca-Cola	45
		Diet Coke	45
Tea (5-ounce cup)		Dr. Pepper	40
1-min. brew	20	Pepsi Cola	38
3-min. brew	35	Diet Pepsi	36
Iced (12 ounces)	70	7 Up	0

increases in their swimming capacity, when the same dose of caffeine was given daily for six weeks, the caffeine caused a significant decrease in swimming capacity.[3]

Chronic caffeine intake is also linked to depression. Caffeine's anti-fatigue and stimulatory effect is largely derived from alteration of the brain's chemistry. Caffeine is a potent blocker of the brain chemical adenosine. Adenosine is like the brain's own Valium. In fact, the way that Valium and similar drugs work is by mimicking the effects of adenosine in the brain. Chronic use of caffeine, by blocking adenosine as well as by altering other chemical processes in the brain, is enough to produce depression and anxiety in some people.

Several studies have found that caffeine intake is extremely high in individuals with psychiatric disorders. The degree of fatigue they experience is often related to how much caffeine they ingest. In one survey of a group of hospitalized psychiatric patients, 61% of those ingesting at least 750 milligrams (5 cups of coffee or more) daily complained of fatigue. Only 54% of those ingesting 250 to 749 milligrams daily, and 24% of those ingesting less than 250 milligrams daily suffered from fatigue.[4]

If, after reading this, you decide to cut back on your caffeine intake, be aware that abrupt cessation of coffee drinking will probably result in symptoms of caffeine withdrawal: fatigue, headache, and an intense desire for coffee.[1,2] Fortunately, this uncomfortable withdrawal period is short-lived.

Drink Green Tea

If you need the occasional burst of energy that caffeine can provide, drink green tea rather than coffee or black tea. Green tea is preferable to black tea because it possesses many important health-promoting properties. Both green tea and black tea are derived from the same plant (*Camellia sinensis*), but green tea is produced by lightly steaming the fresh-cut leaf, while to produce black tea the leaves are allowed to ferment. During fermentation, enzymes present in the tea convert many "polyphenol" substances into "tannins." For green tea, fermentation is not allowed to take place because the prolonged steaming process inactivates these enzymes.

Green tea polyphenols possess phenomenal antioxidant properties and other beneficial effects, including many anti-cancer properties.[5] One key anticancer effect of green tea is its ability to inhibit the formation of the cancer-causing compounds usually ingested with meals. The popular custom of drinking green tea with meals in Japan and China is thought to be a major reason for the low cancer rates in these countries. As the cancer rate in the United States rises, more Americans might want to consider drinking green tea with their meals.

Green tea is relatively low in caffeine content (about 20 to 30 milligrams per 6-ounce cup, depending upon how long it is steeped), but it still can provide the energy boost you may occasionally need, in a much more healthful vehicle.

Refined Carbohydrates and Energy Levels

Dietary carbohydrates are required to provide us with the energy we need for body functions. There are two groups of carbohydrates, simple and complex. Simple carbohydrates, or sugars, are quickly absorbed by the body for a ready source of energy. Many people believe that the assortment of natural, simple sugars in fruits and vegetables have an advantage over sucrose (white sugar) and other refined sugars because they are balanced by a wide range of nutrients that aid in the body's utilization of the sugars. Problems with carbohydrates begin when they are refined and stripped of these nutrients. Virtually all of the vitamin content has been removed from white sugar, white breads and pastries, and many breakfast cereals.

Simple sugars are either monosaccharides composed of one sugar molecule or disaccharides composed of two sugar molecules. The principal monosaccharides that occur in foods are glucose and fructose. The major disaccharides are: sucrose (white sugar) which is composed of one molecule of glucose and one molecule of fructose; maltose (glucose and glucose); and lactose (glucose and galactose).

Glucose is not as sweet-tasting as fructose and sucrose. It is found in abundant amounts in fruits, honey, sweet corn, and most root vegetables. Glucose is also the primary repeating sugar unit of most complex carbohydrates.

Fructose (fruit sugar) is the primary carbohydrate in many fruits, maple syrup, and honey. Fructose is very sweet, roughly one and a half times sweeter than sucrose (white sugar). Although fructose has the same chemical formula as glucose ($C_6H_{12}O_6$), its structure (shape) is quite different. In order to be utilized by the body, fructose must be converted to glucose within the liver.

Complex carbohydrates, or starches, are composed of many simple sugars joined together by chemical bonds. The body breaks down complex carbohydrates into simple sugars gradually, which leads to better blood sugar control. In addition, most complex carbohydrates are good sources of dietary fiber. More and more research indicates that complex carbohydrates should form a major part of the diet. Vegetables, legumes, and grains are excellent sources of complex carbohydrates.

To understand carbohydrates, just remember that eating foods high in simple sugars can be harmful to blood sugar control and energy levels. Always read food labels carefully for clues on sugar content. If the words *sucrose, glucose, maltose, lactose, fructose, corn syrup,* or *white grape juice* concentrate appear on the label, extra sugar has been added.

Currently, more than half of the carbohydrates we consume are in the form of sugars being added to foods as sweetening agents.

Hypoglycemia

Hypoglycemia became a popular diagnosis in the 1970s due to a number of popular books on the subject. *Sugar Blues* by William Duffy, *Hope for Hypoglycemia* by Broda Barnes, and *Sweet and Dangerous* by John Yudkin were among the most popular. The tremendous public interest in hypoglycemia and sugar intake generated by these books and others was met by much skepticism in the medical community. Editorials in the *Journal of the American Medical Association* and *New Journal of Medicine* during that time denounced this popularity and tried to invalidate the existence of hypoglycemia.[6,7]

Presently, an ever-increasing amount of new information on the role that refined carbohydrates and faulty blood sugar control play in many disease processes is emerging. The medical community appears to be finally realizing the important role that refined carbohydrates play in human health and disease. There now exists a substantial amount of information that hypoglycemia and related problems originate from an excess intake of refined carbohydrates.[8–10] While most medical and health organizations (as well as the U.S. government) have recommended that no more than 10% of our total caloric intake be derived from refined sugars added to foods, the fact remains that added sugar accounts for roughly 30% of the total calories consumed by most Americans.[11] The average American consumes over 100 pounds of refined sugar each year. This sugar addiction is part of what is destroying our good health.

Hypoglycemia, Depression, and Chronic Fatigue The most critical nutrient for brain function is glucose or blood sugar. The brain is dependent on glucose as an energy source. When glucose levels are low (as occurs during hypoglycemia), the brain does not function properly and dizziness, headache, clouding of vision, blunted mental acuity, emotional instability, confusion, and abnormal behavior may occur.

The association between hypoglycemia and impaired mental function is well known. Unfortunately, most individuals experiencing depression, anxiety, or other psychological conditions are rarely tested for hypoglycemia, nor are they prescribed a diet which restricts refined carbohydrates.

Numerous studies of depressed individuals have shown a high percentage of hypoglycemia.[12-14] Since depression is one of the most common causes of fatigue, this provides another link between hypoglycemia and chronic fatigue. Simply eliminating refined carbohydrates from the diet is sometimes effective therapy in patients who have depression due to hypoglycemia.

The Glycemic Index   The "glycemic index" was developed by David Jenkins in 1981 to measure the rise of blood glucose after eating a particular food.[15] The standard value of 100 is based on the rise that occurs after the ingestion of glucose. Table 4.2 shows the glycemic index for some common foods. The glycemic index ranges from about 20 for fructose and whole barley to about 98 for a baked potato. Insulin response to carbohydrate-containing foods is similar to the rise in blood sugar.

The glycemic index is used as a dietary guideline for people with either hypoglycemia or diabetes. Basically, people with blood sugar problems should avoid those foods with high values and choose carbohydrate-containing foods with lower values. However, the glycemic index should not be the only dietary guideline. For example, high-fat foods like ice cream and sausage have a low glycemic index because a diet

Table 4.2   Glycemic Index of Some Common Foods[16]

Sugars		Grains (continued)	
Glucose	100	Bread, white	69
Maltose	105	Bread, whole grain	72
Honey	75	Corn	59
Sucrose	60	Corn flakes	80
Fructose	20	Oatmeal	49
Fruits		Pasta	45
Apples	39	Rice	70
Bananas	62	Rice, puffed	95
Oranges	40	Wheat cereal	67
Orange juice	46	*Legumes*	
Raisins	64	Beans	31
Vegetables		Lentils	29
Beets	64	Peas	39
Carrot, raw	31	*Other foods*	
Carrot, cooked	36	Ice cream	36
Potato, baked	98	Milk	34
Potato, boiled	70	Nuts	13
Grains		Sausage	28
Bran cereal	51		

high in fat has been shown to impair glucose tolerance; but obviously these foods are not good choices for people with hypoglycemia or diabetes.

It is interesting to note that fructose has a very low glycemic index. Physicians have historically recommended that individuals with diabetes or hypoglycemia avoid fruits and fructose. Recent research challenges this.[17] Fructose does not cause a rapid rise in blood sugar levels. Because fructose must be changed to glucose in the liver in order to be utilized by the body, blood glucose levels do not rise as rapidly after fructose consumption (compared to other simple sugars). For example, the ingestion of sucrose always results in an immediate elevation in the blood sugar level. Most diabetics and hypoglycemics cannot tolerate sucrose, but most can consume moderate amounts of fruits and fructose without loss of blood sugar control. In fact, fructose and fruits are more easily tolerated than white bread and other refined carbohydrates, and they produce less sharp elevations in blood sugar levels compared to most sources of complex carbohydrates (starch).[18]

Fruits are also excellent sources of many health-promoting substances: vitamin C, carotenes, pectin and other fibers, flavonoids, and polyphenols like ellagic acid. And regular fruit consumption has been shown to offer significant protection against many chronic degenerative diseases including cancer, heart disease, cataracts, and stroke.[10] It simply doesn't make sense to avoid these foods given their important nutritional qualities. Moderation is the key.

Juicing and Good Health   Many medical experts and various departments of the United States government, including the National Academy of Science, the Department of Agriculture, the Department of Health and Human Services, the National Research Council, and the National Cancer Institute, are recommending that Americans consume 2 to 3 servings of fruit and 3 to 5 servings of vegetables per day to help reduce the risk of developing cancer, heart disease, and other chronic degenerative diseases.[10] Unfortunately, less than 10% of the population is meeting even the lowest recommendation—5 servings of a combination of fruits and vegetables.[19]

Juicing is an easy, effective way to meet your body's requirements for fresh fruits and vegetables. Without juicing it is extremely difficult to get the amount of nutrition you need from your foods. Recent studies indicate that to effectively reduce the risk of many cancers, every day we need to eat the amount of beta-carotene in 2 to 3 pounds of fresh carrots (roughly 6 large carrots).[20-23] Just to chew 1 carrot takes 10 or 15 minutes; to eat 6 could take over an hour. Most Americans do not have the desire or the time for this. Juicing is a quick and easy way to meet your daily quota of carotenes and other valuable cancer-fighting nutrients. Sixteen ounces of carrot (or other carotene-rich vegetable) juice provides your body with the carotene found in 3 pounds of carrots, without all the chewing.

It is important to make the juice from fresh fruits and vegetables. Canned, bottled, and frozen juices have been pasteurized or processed in some other manner. As a result, many of the nutritional benefits are already lost.[24-26]

Juicing and Energy Levels   New juice enthusiasts consistently experience a tremendous increase in energy levels. Juicing helps the body's digestive process and allows for quick absorption of high-quality nutrition. The result: more energy. A diet that is rich in raw foods like fresh fruit and vegetable juices reduces stress on the body due to the presence of enzymes in raw foods, the reduced allergenicity of raw foods, and the healthful effect of raw foods on our gut-bacteria ecosystem.

At least half of your diet (by volume or calories) should be composed of raw fruits and vegetables. Juicing is a phenomenal way to reach this goal.

Juicing and Antioxidants   Consuming fresh juices provides the body with high levels of natural plant compounds known as antioxidants. These help protect the body against aging, cancer, heart disease, and many other degenerative conditions by preventing the damaging effects of molecules known as free radicals and pro-oxidants. Although free radicals are produced during normal body processes, our polluted environment increases your free radical load. Cigarette smoking, for example, greatly increases your free radical load. Many of the harmful effects of smoking are related to the extremely high levels of free radicals being inhaled, which deplete key antioxidant nutrients like vitamin C and beta-carotene. Other unhealthy external sources of free radicals include alcohol, fried foods, sunlight, X-rays, many drugs, air pollutants, pesticides, anesthetics, solvents, and formaldehyde. These compounds greatly stress the body's antioxidant mechanisms and may lead to fatigue.

Individuals with chronic fatigue as well as those who are routinely exposed to these factors need antioxidant support. Juicing is an essential part of a dietary program designed to provide optimal levels of antioxidants like carotenes, flavonoids, and chlorophyll; vitamin C, B vitamins, and vitamin E; zinc, manganese, and selenium; and various sulfur-containing compounds, including the amino acids methionine and cysteine.

Designing a Healthful Diet

Most people give little thought to the true nutritional value of their diet. They are motivated to eat foods based on sensual needs rather than what their body requires, or they are "on a diet" to lose weight with little concern for what the body really needs. Health is largely a conscious decision. Awareness of what to eat, in what quantities, and knowing healthy ways to prepare food is critical to our overall health and well-being.

The American Dietetic Association (ADA), in conjunction with the American Diabetes Association and other groups, has developed a diet called the Exchange System, a convenient tool for rapid estimation of the calorie, protein, fat, and carbohydrate content of a diet. Originally created for use in designing dietary recommendations for diabetics, the exchange method is now used in the calculation and design of virtually all therapeutic diets. In my opinion, the ADA exchange plan still does not place a strong enough focus on the quality of food choices.

The Healthy Exchange System presented here is a healthier version because it emphasizes more nutritious food choices and focuses on unprocessed, whole foods. The diet works by allotting a certain number of food exchanges, or servings, per food group each day. There are seven exchange groups, Lists 1 through 7. Lists 6 and 7, the milk and meat groups, are optional, depending on your particular food needs.

The Healthy Exchange System

List 1 Vegetables

List 2 Fruits

List 3 Breads, cereals, and starchy vegetables

List 4 Legumes

List 5 Fats

List 6 Milk

List 7 Meats, fish, cheese, and eggs

Determining Your Caloric Needs

To determine how many calories you need, convert your desirable weight in pounds to kilograms by dividing it by 2.2. Next, take this number and multiply it by the following calories, depending upon your normal activity level:

Little physical activity: 30 calories

Light physical activity: 35 calories

Moderate physical activity: 40 calories

Heavy physical activity: 45 calories

		Number of calories for	Approximate daily calorie
Weight (in kg)	×	activity level	= requirements
_____	×	_____	= _____ calories

Examples of Exchange Recommendations

1,500-Calorie Vegan Diet (daily intake)

List 1 (vegetables)	5 servings
List 2 (fruits)	2 servings
List 3 (breads, cereals, and starchy vegetables)	9 servings
List 4 (legumes)	2½ servings
List 5 (fats)	4 servings

This diet results in an intake of approximately 1,500 calories a day, of which 67% is derived from complex carbohydrates and naturally occurring sugars, 18% from fats, and 15% from proteins. The protein intake is entirely from plant sources, but still provides approximately 55 grams of protein, an amount well above the recommended daily allowance, or RDA, for someone requiring 1,500 calories. At least one-half of the fat servings should be from nuts, seeds, and other whole foods from List 5 of the Healthy Exchange System Lists. The dietary fiber intake is 31 to 74.5 grams. The list that follows summarizes this information.

Percentage of calories as carbohydrates: 67%
Percentage of calories as fats: 18%
Percentage of calories as protein: 15%
Protein content: 55 grams
Dietary fiber content: 31 to 74.5 grams

1,500-Calorie Omnivore Diet (daily intake)

List 1 (vegetables)	5 servings
List 2 (fruits)	2½ servings
List 3 (breads, cereals, and starchy vegetables)	6 servings
List 4 (legumes)	1 serving

List 5 (fats)	5 servings
List 6 (milk)	1 serving
List 7 (meats, fish, cheese, and eggs)	2 servings

Percentage of calories as carbohydrates: 67%
Percentage of calories as fats: 18%
Percentage of calories as protein: 15%
Protein content: 61 grams (75% from plant sources)
Dietary fiber content: 19.5 to 53.5 grams

2,000-Calorie Vegan Diet (daily intake)

List 1 (vegetables)	5½ servings
List 2 (fruits)	2 servings
List 3 (breads, cereals, and starchy vegetables)	11 servings
List 4 (legumes)	5 servings
List 5 (fats)	8 servings

Percentage of calories as carbohydrates: 67%
Percentage of calories as fats: 18%
Percentage of calories as protein: 15%
Protein content: 79 grams
Dietary fiber content: 48.5 to 101.5 grams

2,000-Calorie Omnivore Diet (daily intake)

List 1 (vegetables)	5 servings
List 2 (fruits)	2½ servings
List 3 (breads, cereals, and starchy vegetables)	13 servings
List 4 (legumes)	2 servings
List 5 (fats)	7 servings
List 6 (milk)	1 serving
List 7 (meats, fish, cheese, and eggs)	2 servings

Percentage of calories as carbohydrates: 66%
Percentage of calories as fats: 19%
Percentage of calories as protein: 15%
Protein content: 78 grams (72% from plant sources)
Dietary fiber content: 32.5 to 88.5 grams

2,500-Calorie Vegan Diet (daily intake)

List 1 (vegetables)	8 servings
List 2 (fruits)	3 servings
List 3 (breads, cereals, and starchy vegetables)	17 servings
List 4 (legumes)	5 servings
List 5 (fats)	8 servings

Percentage of calories as carbohydrates: 69%
Percentage of calories as fats: 15%
Percentage of calories as protein: 16%
Protein content: 101 grams
Dietary fiber content: 33 to 121 grams

2,500-Calorie Omnivore Diet (daily intake)

List 1 (vegetables)	8 servings
List 2 (fruits)	3½ servings
List 3 (breads, cereals, and starchy vegetables)	17 servings
List 4 (legumes)	2 servings
List 5 (fats)	8 servings
List 6 (milk)	1 serving
List 7 (meats, fish, cheese, and eggs)	3 servings

Percentage of calories as carbohydrates: 66%
Percentage of calories as fats: 18%
Percentage of calories as protein: 16%

Protein content: 102 grams (80% from plant sources)
Dietary fiber content: 40.5 to 116.5 grams

Note: You may use these diets as the basis for calculating diets of specific caloric amounts. For example, for a 4,000-calorie diet, add the 2,500-calorie diet to the 1,500-calorie diet. For a 1,000-calorie diet, divide the 2,000-calorie diet in half.

The Healthy Exchange System

List 1: Vegetables

Vegetables are an excellent source of vitamins, minerals, and health-promoting fiber compounds. Vegetables are fantastic "diet" foods as they are very high in nutritional value, and low in calories. In addition to eating them whole, vegetables can be consumed as fresh juice. Notice the list of "free" vegetables. These vegetables are termed *free foods* and can be eaten in any desired amount because the calories they contain will be offset by the number of calories your body will burn in the process of digestion. Free foods are especially valuable diet foods because they will keep you feeling satisfied between meals. Please notice that starchy vegetables like potatoes and yams are included in List 3 (breads, cereals, and starchy vegetables).

To meet the Healthy Exchange System's high requirement for vegetable intake many individuals find it easier to juice their fresh, raw vegetables. Juicing allows for easy absorption of the health-giving properties of vegetables in larger amounts.

Vegetables

This list includes the vegetables to use for 1 vegetable serving. Unless otherwise noted, 1 serving consists of 1 cup of cooked vegetables or fresh vegetable juice, or 2 cups of raw vegetables.

Artichoke (1 medium)
Asparagus
Bean sprouts
Beets
Broccoli
Brussels sprouts
Carrots
Cauliflower
Eggplant
Greens
    Beet
    Chard
    Collard
    Dandelion
    Kale
    Mustard
    Spinach
    Turnip
Mushrooms
Okra
Onions
Rhubarb
Rutabaga
Sauerkraut
String beans, green or yellow
Summer squash
Tomatoes, tomato juice, vegetable juice cocktail
Zucchini

Free vegetables
Eat as many of the following items as you wish.

Alfalfa sprouts
Bell peppers
Bok choy
Cabbage
Celery
Chicory
Chinese cabbage
Cucumber
Endive
Escarole
Lettuce
Parsley
Radishes
Spinach
Turnips
Watercress

List 2: Fruits

Fruits make excellent snacks as they contain fructose or fruit sugar which is absorbed slowly into the bloodstream, allowing the body sufficient time to utilize it. Fruits are also excellent sources of vitamins and minerals as well as health-promoting fiber compounds and flavonoids. Fruits are not as nutrient-dense as vegetables, because they are typically higher in calories. That is why vegetables are favored over fruits in weight-loss plans and overall healthful diets.

Fruits
Each of the following equals 1 serving.

Fresh fruit and fruit-based items
Fresh juice, 1 cup (8 ounces)*
Pasteurized juice, ⅔ cup

Apple, 1 large
Applesauce (unsweetened), 1 cup
Apricots, dried, 8 halves
Apricots, fresh, 4 medium
Banana, 1 medium
Berries
    Blackberries, 1 cup
    Blueberries, 1 cup
    Cranberries, 1 cup
    Raspberries, 1 cup
    Strawberries, 1½ cups
Cherries, 20 large
Dates, 4
Figs, dried, 2
Figs, fresh, 2
Grapefruit, 1
Grapes, 20
Mango, 1 small
Melons
    Cantaloupe, ½ small
    Honeydew, ¼ medium
    Watermelon, 2 cups
Nectarine, 2 small
Orange, 1 large
Papaya, 1½ cups
Peaches, 2 medium
Persimmons, native, 2 medium
Pineapple, 1 cup

Plums, 4 medium

Prune juice, ½ cup

Prunes, 4 medium

Raisins, 4 tablespoons

Tangerine, 2 medium

Processed fruit and other products

Eat no more than 1 serving per day.

Honey, 1 tablespoon

Jams, jellies, preserves, 1 tablespoon

Sugar, 1 tablespoon

*Although 1 cup of most fruit juices equals 1 serving, ½ cup of prune juice will suffice.

List 3: Breads, Cereals, and Starchy Vegetables

Breads, cereals, and starchy vegetables are classified as complex carbohydrates. Complex carbohydrates are made up of long chains of simple carbohydrates, or sugars. This means the human body has to digest, or break down, the large sugar chains into simple sugars. Therefore, the sugar from complex carbohydrates enters the bloodstream slowly. A relatively stable blood sugar level and appetite is the result.

Complex carbohydrates—breads, cereals, and starchy vegetables—are higher in fiber and nutrients and lower in calories than simple-sugar items such as cakes and candies.

Breads, Cereals, and Starchy Vegetables

Each of the following items equals 1 serving.

Breads

Bagel, small, ½

Dinner roll, 1

Dried bread crumbs, 3 tablespoons

English muffin, small, ½

Tortilla (6-inch), 1

Whole wheat, rye, or pumpernickel, 1 slice

Cereals

Bran flakes, ½ cup

Cornmeal (dry), 2 tablespoons

Flour, 2½ tablespoons

Grits (cooked), ½ cup

Pasta (cooked), ½ cup

Porridge (cooked cereal), ½ cup

Puffed cereal (unsweetened), 1 cup

Rice or barley (cooked), ½ cup

Unpuffed unsweetened cereal, ¾ cup

Wheat germ, ¼ cup

Crackers

Arrowroot, 3

Graham (2½-inch squares), 2

Matzo (4 by 6 inches), ½

Rye wafers (2 by 3½ inches), 3

Saltine, 6

Starchy vegetables

Corn, kernel, ⅓ cup

Corn on the cob, 1 small

Parsnips, ⅔ cup

Potato, mashed, ½ cup

Potato, white, 1 small

Squash (acorn, butternut, or winter), ½ cup

Yam or sweet potato, ¼ cup

Prepared foods

Each of the following items equals 1 "bread" serving, but you must omit 1 or more fat servings to maintain the nutrition balance of your diet.

Biscuit, 2-inch diameter, 1 (omit 1 fat serving)
Corn bread, 2 by 2 by 1 inch, 1 (omit 1 fat serving)
French fries, 2 to 3 inches long, 8 (omit 1 fat serving)
Muffin, small, 1 (omit 1 fat serving)
Pancake, 5 by ½ inch, 1 (omit 1 fat serving)
Potato or corn chips, 15 (omit 2 fat servings)
Waffle, 5 by ½ inch, 1 (omit 1 fat serving)

List 4: Legumes

According to the dictionary, a legume is a plant that produces a pod that splits on both sides. Of the common human foods, beans, peas, lentils, and peanuts are legumes. The legume category also includes alfalfa, clover, acacia, and indigo. Legumes are fantastic foods as they are rich in important nutrients and health-promoting compounds. Legumes help improve liver function, lower cholesterol levels, and are extremely effective in improving blood sugar control. Since obesity and diabetes have been linked to loss of blood sugar control (insulin insensitivity), legumes appear to be extremely important in weight-loss plans and in the dietary management of diabetes.

Legumes

In this list, ½ cup of each item, cooked or sprouted, equals 1 serving.

Black-eyed peas
Chickpeas
Garbanzo beans
Kidney beans
Lentils
Lima beans
Pinto beans

Soybeans, including tofu (omit 1 fat serving)
Split peas
Other dried beans and peas

List 5: Fats and Oils

Animal fats are typically solid at room temperature and are referred to as saturated fats, while vegetable fats are liquid at room temperature and are referred to as unsaturated fats, or oils. Vegetable oils provide the greatest source of the essential fatty acids linoleic acid and linolenic acid. These fatty acids function in our bodies as components of nerve cells, cellular membranes, and hormone-like substances. Fats also provide the body with energy.

While fats are important to human health, too much fat in the diet, especially saturated fat, is linked to numerous cancers, heart disease, and stroke. Most nutritional experts recommend that your total fat intake be less than 30% of your total calories, and that you consume at least twice as much unsaturated fat as saturated fat.

Fats and Oils
Each of the following equals 1 serving.

Mono-unsaturated
Olive oil, 1 teaspoon
Olives, 5 small

Polyunsaturated
Almonds, 10 whole
Avocado (4-inch diameter), ⅛ fruit
Peanuts
　　Spanish, 20 whole
　　Virginia, 10 whole

Pecans, 2 large
Seeds
    Flax, 1 tablespoon
    Pumpkin, 1 tablespoon
    Sesame, 1 tablespoon
    Sunflower, 1 tablespoon
Vegetable oil
    Canola, 1 teaspoon
    Corn, 1 teaspoon
    Flaxseed, 1 teaspoon
    Safflower, 1 teaspoon
    Soy, 1 teaspoon
    Sunflower, 1 teaspoon
Walnuts, 6 small

Saturated (use sparingly)
Bacon, 1 slice
Butter, 1 teaspoon
Cream, heavy, 1 tablespoon
Cream, light or sour, 2 tablespoons
Cream cheese, 1 tablespoon
Mayonnaise, 1 teaspoon
Salad dressing, 2 teaspoons

List 6: Milk

Is milk for everybody? Definitely not. Many people are allergic to milk or lack the enzymes necessary to digest it. The drinking of cow's milk is a relatively new dietary practice for humans. This may be the reason so many people have difficulty with milk. Certainly milk consumption should be limited to no more than two servings per day.

Milk

For each of the following items, 1 cup equals 1 "milk" serving, but for some items you must omit 1 or more fat servings to maintain the nutrition balance of your diet.

Nonfat milk or yogurt
Nonfat soy milk
2% milk or soy milk (omit 1 fat serving)
Lowfat yogurt (omit 1 fat serving)
Whole milk (omit 2 fat servings)
Yogurt (omit 2 fat servings)

List 7: Meats, Fish, Cheese, and Eggs

When choosing from this list, choose primarily from the lowfat group and remove the skin of poultry. This practice will keep the amount of saturated fat low. Although many people advocate vegetarianism, List 7 provides high concentrations of certain nutrients difficult to get in an entirely vegetarian diet. It provides the full range of amino acids, vitamin B12, and iron. Nonetheless, if you have any inflammatory condition, it is best to avoid the meat food group (with the exception of cold-water fish).

Meats, Fish, Cheese, and Eggs
Each of the following items equals 1 serving.

Lowfat items
Beef, 1 ounce
> Baby beef, chipped beef, chuck, round (bottom, top), rump (all cuts), steak (flank, plate), spareribs, tenderloin plate ribs, tripe

Cottage cheese, lowfat, ¼ cup
Fish, 1 ounce

Lamb, 1 ounce

> Leg, loin (roast and chops), ribs, shank, sirloin, shoulder

Poultry (chicken or turkey without skin), 1 ounce

Veal, 1 ounce

> Cutlet, leg, loin, rib, shank, shoulder

Medium-fat items

For each of the following items, omit ½ fat serving.

Beef, 1 ounce

> Canned corned beef, ground (15% fat), rib eye, round (ground commercial)

Cheese, 1 ounce

> Farmer, Mozzarella, Parmesan, ricotta

Eggs, 1

Organ meats, 1 ounce

Peanut butter, 2 tablespoons

Pork, 1 ounce

> Boiled, Boston butt, Canadian bacon, loin (all tenderloin), picnic

High-fat items

For each of the following items, omit 2 fat servings.

Beef, 1 ounce

> Brisket, corned beef, ground beef (more than 20% fat), hamburger, roasts (rib), steaks (club and rib)

Cheese, cheddar, 1 ounce

Duck or goose, 1 ounce

Lamb, breast, 1 ounce

Pork, 1 ounce

> Country-style ham, deviled ham, ground pork, loin, spareribs

Menu Planning

The Healthy Exchange System was created to ensure that you are consuming a diet that provides adequate nutrients in their proper ratio. Once you have determined your caloric needs and have calculated the number of servings you require from each Healthy Exchange List, construct a daily menu plan and follow it.

Breakfast

Breakfast is an absolute must. Healthful breakfast choices include whole-grain cereals, muffins, and breads, along with fresh whole fruit or fresh fruit juice. Cereals, both hot and cold, preferably from whole grains, are among the best food choices for breakfast. The complex carbohydrates in the grains provide sustained energy. Also, an evaluation of data from the National Health and Nutrition Examination Survey II (a national survey of the nutritional and health practices of Americans) disclosed that serum cholesterol levels are lowest among adults who eat whole-grain cereal for breakfast.[27] Individuals who consumed other breakfast foods had high blood cholesterol levels, and levels were highest among those who typically skipped breakfast.

Lunch

Lunch is a great time to enjoy a nourishing bowl of soup, a large salad, and some whole-grain bread. Bean soups and other legume dishes are especially good lunch selections for people with diabetes and blood sugar problems, due to their ability to improve blood sugar regulation. Legumes are filling, yet low in calories.

Snacks

The best snacks are nuts, seeds, and fresh fruits and vegetables (including fresh fruit and vegetable juices).

Dinner

For dinner, the healthiest meals will contain a fresh vegetable salad, a cooked vegetable side dish or a bowl of soup, whole grains, and legumes. The whole grains may be provided in bread, pasta, as a side dish, or part of a recipe for an entrée. Legumes can be utilized in soups, salads, and main dishes. Although a mixed, varied diet rich in whole grains, vegetables, and legumes can provide optimal levels of protein, many people like to eat meat. The important thing is not to overconsume animal products. Limit your intake to no more than 4 to 6 ounces per day and choose fish, skinless poultry, and lean cuts rather than fatty meats.

Finding and Controlling Food Allergies

In addition to following the guidelines of the Healthy Exchange System, people with chronic fatigue should consider the possible influence of food allergies (see Chapter 2). Once a food allergy has been determined, the simplest, most effective method of dealing with it will be by avoiding the offending food. Avoidance means not eating the food in its most identifiable state (eggs in an omelet), or in its hidden state (eggs in bread). Closely related foods with similar components may also need to be eliminated (for example, rice and millet in patients with severe wheat allergy).

It will also be important to eliminate food additives. Food additives are used to prevent spoiling or enhance flavor and include such substances as preservatives, artificial colors, artificial flavorings, and acidifiers. Food additives are linked to allergies as well as depression, asthma, hyperactivity or learning disabilities in children, and migraine headaches.[28]

If a person has multiple food allergies, the so-called rotary diversified diet is the best method to follow. This diet is made up of a highly varied selection of foods which are eaten in a definite rotation, in order to prevent the formation of new allergies and to control pre-existing ones. Tolerated foods are eaten at regularly spaced intervals of four to seven days. For example, if a person has wheat on Monday, they will have to wait until Friday to have anything with wheat in it again. This approach is based on the principle that infrequent consumption of tolerated foods is not likely to induce new allergies or increase any mild allergies. As tolerance for eliminated foods returns, that food may be added back into the rotation schedule without reactivation of the allergy. (This of course applies only to cyclic food allergies—fixed allergenic foods may never be eaten again.)

Besides rotating tolerated foods, food families must also be rotated. All foods, whether animal or vegetable, come in families, and foods in one family can "cross-react" with allergy-inducing foods. Steady consumption of foods which are members of the same family can lead to allergies. Food families need not be as strictly rotated as individual foods. I usually recommend avoiding members of the same food family two days in a row. Table 4.3 lists family classifications for edible plants and animals. A simplified four-day rotation diet plan is provided in Table 4.4.

Chapter Summary

Individuals who suffer from chronic fatigue need supernutrition. They need high-quality foods for fuel and they will want to avoid foods which rob the body of energy. To repeat the basic dietary recommendations in this chapter:

1. Eliminate or restrict the intake of caffeine.
2. Eliminate refined carbohydrates.
3. Buy and use a juicer.
4. Design a healthful diet.
5. Eat regular, planned meals.
6. Rotate foods to prevent food allergies.

Table 4.3 Edible Plant and Animal Kingdom Taxonomic List

Vegetables

Legumes	**Mustard**	**Parsley**	**Potato**
Beans	Broccoli	Anise	Chile
Cocoa beans	Brussels sprouts	Caraway	Eggplant
Lentils	Cabbage	Carrot	Peppers
Licorice	Cauliflower	Celery	Potatoes
Peanuts	Mustard	Coriander	Tobacco
Peas	Radish	Cumin	Tomato
Soybeans	Turnip	Parsley	
Tamarinds	Watercress		
Grass	**Lily**	**Laurel**	**Sunflower**
Barley	Asparagus	Avocado	Artichoke
Corn	Chives	Camphor	Lettuce
Oat	Garlic	Cinnamon	Sunflower
Rice	Leeks		
Rye	Onions		
Wheat			
Beet	**Buckwheat**		
Beet	Buckwheat		
Chard	Rhubarb		
Spinach			

Fruits

Gourds	**Plums**	**Citrus**	**Cashew**
Cantaloupe	Almond	Grapefruit	Cashews
Cucumber	Apricot	Lemon	Mango
Honeydew	Cherry	Lime	Pistachio
Melons	Peach	Mandarin	
Pumpkin	Persimmon	Orange	
Squash	Plum	Tangerine	
Zucchini			

Table 4.3   *(continued)*

Fruits (cont.)

Nuts	Beech	Banana	Palm
Brazil nuts	Beechnuts	Arrowroot	Coconut
Pecans	Chestnuts	Banana	Date
Walnuts	Chinquapin nuts	Plantain	Date sugar

Grape	Pineapple	Rose	Birch
Grape	Pineapple	Blackberry	Filberts
Raisin		Loganberry	Hazelnuts
		Raspberry	
		Rose hips	
		Strawberry	

Apple	Blueberry	Pawpaws
Apple	Blueberry	Papaya
Pear	Cranberry	Pawpaw
Quince	Huckleberry	

Animals

Mammals (Meat/Milk)	Birds (Meat/Egg)	Fish	
Cow	Chicken	Catfish	Salmon
Goat	Duck	Cod	Sardine
Pig	Goose	Flounder	Snapper
Rabbit	Hen	Halibut	Trout
Sheep	Turkey	Mackerel	Tuna

Crustaceans	Mollusks
Crab	Abalone
Crayfish	Clams
Lobster	Mussels
Prawn	Oysters
Shrimp	Scallops

*The names of food families are shown in this table in boldface.

Table 4.4 Four-day Rotation Diet

Food Family	Food
Day 1	
Citrus	Lemon, orange, grapefruit, lime, tangerine, kumquat, citron
Banana	Banana, plantain, arrowroot (musa)
Palm	Coconut, date, date sugar
Parsley	Carrots, parsnips, celery, celery seed, celeriac, anise, dill, fennel, cumin, parsley, coriander, caraway
Spices	Black and white pepper, peppercorn, nutmeg, mace
Subucaya	Brazil nut
Bird	All fowl and game birds, including chicken, turkey, duck, goose, guinea, pigeon, quail, pheasant, eggs
Juices	Juices (preferably fresh) may be made and used from any fruits and vegetables listed above, in any combination desired, without adding sweeteners.
Day 2	
Grape	All varieties of grapes, raisins
Pineapple	Juice-pack, water-pack, or fresh
Rose	Strawberry, raspberry, blackberry, loganberry, rose hips
Gourd	Watermelon, cucumber, cantaloupe, pumpkin, squash, other melons, zucchini, pumpkin or squash seeds
Beet	Beet, spinach, chard
Legume	Peas, black-eyed peas, dry beans, green beans, carob, soybeans, lentils, licorice, peanuts, alfalfa
Cashew	Cashew, pistachio, mango
Birch	Filberts, hazelnuts
Flaxseed	Flaxseed
Swine	All pork products
Mollusks	Abalone, snail, squid, clam, mussel, oyster, scallop
Crustaceans	Crab, crayfish, lobster, prawn, shrimp
Juices	Juices (preferably fresh) may be made and used without added sweeteners from any fruits, berries, or vegetables listed above, in any combination desired, including fresh alfalfa and some legumes.

Table 4.4   *(continued)*

Food Family	Food
Day 3	
Apple	Apple, pear, quince
Gooseberry	Currant, gooseberry
Buckwheat	Buckwheat, rhubarb
Aster	Lettuce, chicory, endive, escarole, globe artichoke, dandelion, sunflower seeds, tarragon
Potato	Potato, tomato, eggplant, peppers (red and green), chile pepper, paprika, cayenne, ground cherries
Lily (onion)	Onion, garlic, asparagus, chives, leeks
Spurge	Tapioca
Herb	Basil, savory, sage, oregano, horehound, catnip, spearmint, peppermint, thyme, marjoram, lemon balm
Walnut	English walnut, black walnut, pecan, hickory nut, butternut
Pedalium	Sesame
Beech	Chestnut
Saltwater fish	Herring, anchovy, cod, sea bass, sea trout, mackerel, tuna, swordfish, flounder, sole
Freshwater fish	Sturgeon, salmon, whitefish, bass, perch
Juices	Juices (preferably fresh) may be made and used without added sweeteners from any fruits and vegetables listed above, in any combination.
Day 4	
Plum	Plum, cherry, peach, apricot, nectarine, almond, wild cherry
Blueberry	Blueberry, huckleberry, cranberry, wintergreen
Pawpaws	Pawpaw, papaya, papain
Mustard	Mustard, turnip, radish, horseradish, watercress, cabbage, Chinese cabbage, broccoli, cauliflower, Brussels sprouts, kale, kohlrabi, rutabaga
Laurel	Avocado, cinnamon, bay leaf, sassafras, cassia buds or bark
Sweet potato or yam	

Table 4.4   *(continued)*

Food Family	Food
Day 4 (cont.)	
Grass	Wheat, corn, rice, oats, barley, rye, wild rice, cane, millet, sorghum, bamboo sprouts
Orchid	Vanilla
Protea	Macadamia nut
Conifer	Pine nut
Fungus	Mushrooms and yeast (brewer's yeast, etc.)
Bovid	Milk products—butter, cheese, yogurt, beef and milk products, oleomargarine, lamb
Juices	Juices (preferably fresh) may be made and used without added sweeteners from any fruits and vegetables listed above, in any combination desired.

5

Physical Care of the Body

A critical component in the energy equation is the physical status of the body. You may recall reading in Chapter 3 that how energetic you feel at any given time is dependent upon a combination of two simple factors: what your mind is focusing on and your physiology. Physiology includes not only the chemicals and hormones floating around in your body, but also your posture, degree of muscle tension, and your breathing.

This chapter focuses on the physical care of the body to produce higher energy levels. The physical care of the human body involves the following four areas:

> Breathing
> Posture
> Bodywork
> Exercise

Breathing

Have you ever noticed how a baby breathes? With each breath the abdomen rises and falls because the baby is breathing with its diaphragm. If you are like most adults, you tend to fill only your upper chest because you do not utilize the diaphragm. Shallow breathing tends to produce tension and fatigue. I have yet to see a patient with chronic fatigue who was not also a shallow (chest-only) breather.

One of the most powerful methods of producing more energy and less stress in the body is by breathing with the diaphragm. Try it. Take in a deep, natural breath by using your diaphragm and let it out slowly. By using your diaphragm to breathe, you dramatically change your physiology. Learn what it feels like to breathe easily and naturally using your diaphragm and you will definitely notice improved energy levels, reduced tension, and improved mental alertness.

Posture

Most people with chronic fatigue are in a posture, whether sitting or standing, that tends to reinforce fatigue. The manner in which the body is held usually reflects energy levels. When the body is slouched, shoulders slumped, and head down, diaphragmatic breathing is more difficult. Poor posture promotes shallow breathing and low energy levels. Notice (standing or sitting) that when you breathe with the diaphragm, it changes your posture to expand the chest cavity. As a result of good diaphragmatic breathing, the spine becomes more erect, the shoulders are pushed back, and the head is pulled up. Energetic posture and good diaphragmatic breathing usually go hand in hand.

To get more energy moving in your body, assume more energetic postures. It sends a message to the subconscious that you are energized and ready to go. Become aware of how you are holding your body as well as how you are breathing.

If you have chronic fatigue, you probably tend to have poor posture, head slightly down, shoulders slouched. When you find yourself in this position, start breathing with your diaphragm and pull your head up—imagine a cord at the top of your head gently pulling your spine and neck straight and into alignment.

If you notice a great deal of muscular tension or stress in your body, the next phase of physical care of the body comes into play—bodywork.

Bodywork

The need to touch and be touched is universal. Around the world, bodywork practitioners are relied upon much more than in the United States. However, there is a growing trend toward bodywork treatments by Americans.

Many different types of bodywork can provide benefits to individuals with chronic fatigue: Various massage techniques, chiropractic spinal adjustment and manipulation, Rolfing, reflexology, shiatsu, and many more of these techniques can work. It is really a matter of personal preference. Finding a technique or practitioner who you really like and incorporating bodywork into your routine can make a world of difference.

I have experienced a broad range of bodywork, from Rolfing and deep-tissue massage (often referred to as a sport massage) to more gentle techniques like craniosacral therapy and Trager massage. I have learned that the therapist is more critical to the outcome than the technique; the technique is only a tool. Depending on the person, my own experience has been that deep-tissue work like Rolfing and Hellerwork are the most powerful bodywork techniques to create changes in body posture and energy levels.

Unlike basic massage and chiropractic spinal adjustment, which focus on the muscles and spine, Rolfing and Hellerwork work with the elastic sheathing network that helps support the body and keeps bones, muscles, and organs in place. This network is known as the fascia. Rolfers and Hellerwork practitioners believe that the fascia can be damaged by physical injury, emotional trauma, and bad postural habits. The body is thrown out of alignment. Rolfing, Hellerwork, and other deep-tissue treatments attempt to bring the body back into balance, restore efficiency of movement, and increase mobility by stretching and lengthening the fascia, returning it to its natural form and pliability.

Rolfing or Hellerwork treatments consist of ten or eleven sessions, each lasting between 60 and 90 minutes. Treatments are sequential, beginning with more superficial treatments and ending with deeper massage. You should know that deep-tissue treatment can be quite painful, but the rewards are worth it: improved breathing, posture, tolerance to stress, and, of course, higher energy levels. In addition, many people going through deep-tissue therapy like Rolfing and Hellerwork report resolution of emotional conflicts. It seems that many painful or traumatic experiences are stored in the fascia and muscles as tension. Releasing the tension and restoring freedom in the fascia can produce remarkable increases in energy levels.

If Rolfing or Hellerwork is too painful for you, there is a light-touch therapy that feels incredibly pleasurable that I think can produce similar, but more gradual, results. The technique is called Tragerwork or Trager massage, the innovation of Milton Trager, M.D. According to Trager, we all develop mental and physical patterns that may limit our movements or contribute to fatigue as well as pain and tension. During a typical session, the practitioner gently and rhythmically rocks, cradles, and moves the body and encourages the client to see that freedom of movement and relaxation are entirely possible. The aim of the treatment is not so much to massage or manipulate, but rather to promote feelings of lightness, freedom, and well-being. Clients are also taught a series of exercises to do at home. Called Mentastics, these simple, dance-like movements are designed to help maintain and enhance the feelings of flexibility and freedom that were experienced during the sessions.

Exercise

Bodywork alone is not enough to promote good health. Our bodies really require more intense movements and the benefits of regular exercise. The immediate effect of exercise is stress on the body, however, with a regular exercise program the body adapts. The body's response to this regular stress is that it becomes stronger, functions more efficiently, and has greater endurance. Exercise is a vital component of health.

Physical Benefits of Exercise   The entire body benefits from regular exercise, largely as a result of improved cardiovascular and respiratory function. Simply stated, exercise enhances the transport of oxygen and nutrients into cells. At the same time, exercise enhances the transport of carbon dioxide and waste products from the tissues of the body to the bloodstream and ultimately to eliminative organs.

Regular exercise is particularly beneficial in reducing the risk of heart disease. It does this by lowering cholesterol levels, increasing blood and oxygen supply to the heart, inproving the functional capacity of the heart, reducing blood pressure, reducing obesity, and exerting a favorable effect on blood clotting.[1]

Regular exercise increases stamina and energy levels. People who exercise regularly are much less likely to suffer from fatigue and depression.

Psychological and Social Benefits of Exercise   Tension, depression, feelings of inadequacy, and worries tend to diminish with regular exercise. Exercise alone has been demonstrated to have a tremendous impact on improving mood and the ability to handle stressful life situations.

In a study published in the *American Journal of Epidemiology*, it was found that increased participation in exercise, sports, and physical activities is strongly associated with decreased symptoms of depression (feelings that life is not worthwhile, low spirits), anxiety (restlessness, tension), and malaise (rundown feeling, insomnia).[2]

Exercise and Immune Function

In addition to the benefits cited above, regular exercise has also been shown to lead to improved immune status. In regards to CFS, regular exercise has been shown to lead to significant increase (up to 100%) in natural killer cell activity.[3,4] Although strenuous exercise is required to benefit the cardiovascular system, light to moderate exercise may be best for the immune system. One study found that immune function was significantly increased by the practice of Tai Chi exercises.[5] Tai Chi is a martial art that features movement from one posture to the next in a flowing motion that resembles a slow dance. The research thus far suggests that light to moderate exercise stimulates the immune system, while intense exercise (like training for the Olympics) can have the opposite effect.[6]

Designing an Exercise Program

The first thing to do is to make sure you are fit enough to start an exercise program. If you have been mostly inactive for a number of years or have a previously diagnosed illness, please consult your physician first.

If you are declared fit enough to begin, the next thing to do is select an activity that you would enjoy. The best exercises are the kind that get your heart moving. Aerobic activities such as walking briskly, jogging, bicycling, cross-country skiing, swimming, aerobic dance, and racquet sports are good examples. Brisk walking (5 miles an hour) for approximately 30 minutes may be the very best form of exercise for weight loss. Walking can be done anywhere; it doesn't require any expensive equipment, just comfortable clothing and well-fitting shoes; and the risk for injury is extremely low.

Exercise draws from all of the fat stores of the body, not just from local deposits of the body parts being used. While aerobic exercise generally enhances weight-loss programs, weight-training programs can also substantially alter body composition by increasing lean body weight and decreasing body fat. Thus weight training may be just as effective as aerobic exercise in maintaining or increasing lean body weight.

Intensity   Exercise intensity is determined by measuring your heart rate (the number of times your heart beats per minute). This can be done by placing the index and middle finger of one hand on the side of the neck just below the angle of the jaw, or on the opposite wrist. Beginning with zero, count the number of heartbeats for 6 seconds. Simply add a zero to this number and you have your pulse. For example, if you counted 14 beats, your heart rate is 140. Is this a good number? It depends upon your "training zone."

A quick and easy way to determine your maximum training heart rate is to subtract your age from 185. For example, if you are 40 years old, your maximum heart rate would be 145. To determine the bottom of the training zone, simply subtract 20 from this number. In the case of a 40-year-old this would be 125. So, your training range would be a heartbeat between 125 and 145 beats per minute. For maximum health benefits you must stay in this range and never exceed it.

Duration and Frequency   A minimum of 15 to 20 minutes of exercise at your training heart rate at least three times a week is necessary to gain any significant cardiovascular benefits from exercise. It is better to exercise at the lower end of your training zone for longer periods of time than it is to exercise at a higher intensity for a shorter period of time. It works best if you can make light exercise a part of your daily routine.

Fun   The key to getting the maximum benefit from exercise is to make it enjoyable. Choose an activity that you enjoy and is fun. If you can take pleasure from exercise, you are much more likely to exercise regularly. You don't get in good physical condition by exercising once, it must happen on a regular basis. So you might as well make it fun.

Chapter Summary

Proper care of the body is critical to high energy levels. Breathing with the diaphragm, good posture, bodywork, and regular exercise all help to relieve tensions that can pull down your energy levels. Taking good physical care of yourself is one of the best methods for changing your physiology and producing higher energy levels.

6

Nutritional Supplementation

In the last few years more Americans than ever are taking nutritional supplements.[1] Tremendous scientific evidence supports the use of vitamins and minerals as an aid to optimal health. While severe nutritional deficiencies are uncommon in the United States, there is evidence that "subclinical" or marginal deficiency is common.[2] A subclinical deficiency indicates a deficiency of a particular vitamin or mineral that is not severe enough to produce a classic deficiency sign or symptom. Complicating the matter, in many instances the only clue of a subclinical nutrient deficiency may be fatigue, lethargy, difficulty in concentration, a lack of well-being, or some other vague symptom. Diagnosis of subclinical deficiencies is an extremely difficult process that involves detailed dietary or laboratory analysis.

Scientific research overwhelmingly indicates that the optimal level for many nutrients, especially the so-called antioxidant nutrients like vitamins C and E, beta-carotene, and selenium, may be much higher than their current recommended daily allowance (RDA). The RDAs focus only on the prevention of nutritional deficiencies in population groups, they do not define optimal intake for an individual.[3]

Multiple Vitamin-Mineral Formulas

Many Americans look to multiple vitamin and mineral supplements as a way to increase their intake of essential nutrients. To highlight the potential benefits of taking a multiple vitamin-mineral supplement to improve your health, vitality, and body function, let's examine the results of a recent study of the effect of nutritional supplementation on immune function.

The study was double-blind—one group received a multiple vitamin and mineral formula, the other group received an identical-looking placebo.[4] Results of the twelve-month study indicated that subjects taking the real nutritional supplements demonstrated improvements in many immune system parameters and had significantly fewer infections compared to the placebo group. This study highlights the essential role that nutrition plays in maintaining a healthy immune system (discussed further in Chapter 8). A deficiency of virtually any nutrient will result in impaired immune system function.

A subclinical vitamin and mineral deficiency may be responsible for the impaired immune function in many patients suffering from CFS. The closer an individual's essential nutrient intake is to being optimal, the better chance he or she has that the immune system will function in an optimal manner.

A Quick Guide to Vitamins and Minerals

Thirteen different vitamins are known, each with its own special role to play. The vitamins are classified into two groups: fat-soluble (A, D, E, and K) and water-soluble (the B vitamins and vitamin C). Vitamins function along with enzymes in chemical reactions necessary for human bodily function, including energy production. Vitamins and enzymes act together as catalysts in speeding up the making or breaking of chemical bonds that join molecules together.

Twenty-two different minerals are important in human nutrition. Like vitamins, minerals function as components of body enzymes. Minerals are also needed for proper composition of bones and blood, and help maintain normal cell function.

This book is full of examples of the ways in which certain body functions can be significantly improved by supplementing the diet with a specific vitamin or mineral. However, good health requires a strong foundation. The recommendations in Table 6.1 for daily intake levels of vitamins and minerals are designed to provide an optimum intake range for maintaining health. These recommended levels are most easily attained by taking a good multiple vitamin-mineral formula and then adding specific nutrients, like vitamin C and beta-carotene, as needed.

Special Nutrients for Chronic Fatigue

Several nutrients deserve special consideration if you are suffering from chronic fatigue: vitamin C, magnesium, and iron. In addition, liver extracts have been shown to have beneficial effects.

Vitamin C

The primary function of vitamin C is the manufacture of collagen, the main protein substance of the human body. Collagen is an important protein for the structures that hold our body together (connective tissue, cartilage, tendons), and

Table 6.1   Daily Optimal Supplementation Range for Adults

Vitamins	Daily Dosage
Vitamin A (retinol)	5,000–10,000 IU*
Vitamin A (from beta-carotene)	10,000–75,000 IU
Vitamin D	100–400 IU
Vitamin E (d-alpha tocopherol)	400–1,200 IU
Vitamin K (phytonadione)	60–900 mcg†
Vitamin C (ascorbic acid)	500–9,000 mg
Vitamin B1 (thiamine)	10–90 mg
Vitamin B2 (riboflavin)	10–90 mg
Niacin	10–90 mg
Niacinamide	10–30 mg
Vitamin B6 (pyridoxine)	25–100 mg
Biotin	100–300 mcg
Pantothenic acid	25–100 mg
Folic acid	400–1,000 mcg
Vitamin B12	400–1,000 mcg
Choline	150–500 mg
Inositol	150–500 mg
Minerals	
Boron	1–2 mg
Calcium	250–750 mg
Chromium	200–400 mcg
Copper	1–2 mg
Iodine	50–150 mcg
Iron	15–30 mg
Magnesium	500–750 mg
Manganese	10–15 mg
Molybdenum	10–25 mcg
Potassium	200–500 mg
Selenium	100–200 mcg
Silica	200–1,000 mcg
Vanadium	50–100 mcg
Zinc	15–30 mg

*IU = International Units
†mcg = microgram

vitamin C is vital for wound repair, healthy gums, and the prevention of easy bruising. In scurvy or severe vitamin C deficiency, the classic symptoms are bleeding gums, poor wound healing, and excessive bruising. Susceptibility to infection, hysteria, and depression are also hallmark features.[5] In addition to its role in collagen metabolism, vitamin C is also critical to immune function, the manufacture of certain nerve-transmitting substances and hormones, and the absorption and utilization of other nutrients. Vitamin C is a very important nutritional antioxidant as well.[5]

Numerous experimental, clinical, and population studies have shown that increasing your intake of vitamin C will have a number of beneficial effects:

Reduces your risk of cancer

Boosts the immune system

Protects against pollution and cigarette smoke

Enhances wound repair

Increases life expectancy

Reduces the risk of cataracts[6]

Many claims have been made about the role of vitamin C in boosting the immune system, especially in regards to the prevention and treatment of the common cold. However, despite numerous positive clinical and experimental studies this effect is still hotly debated.[6,7] From a biochemical viewpoint, there is considerable evidence that vitamin C plays a vital role in many immune mechanisms. The high concentration of vitamin C in white blood cells, particularly lymphocytes, is rapidly depleted during infection, and a relative vitamin C deficiency may ensue if vitamin C is not regularly replenished.[6]

Vitamin C has been shown to benefit many different immune functions including enhancing white blood cell function and activity; and increasing interferon levels, antibody responses, antibody levels, secretion of thymic hormones, and integrity of ground substance.[5,6] Vitamin C also possesses many biochemical effects very similar to interferon, the body's natural antiviral and anticancer compound.[8]

During times of chemical, emotional, psychological, or physiological stress, the urinary excretion of vitamin C is increased, signifying an increased need for vitamin C during these times.[6,9] Examples of chemical stressors include cigarette smoke, pollutants, and allergens. Vitamin C supplements, along with an increased intake of vitamin C-rich foods, is often recommended to keep the immune system working properly during times of stress.[9] Other conditions where extra vitamin C is often recommended include infections, allergies, cataracts, high cholesterol, high blood pressure, diabetes, and hepatitis.

The debate over how much vitamin C is optimum is an ongoing one. At one end of the spectrum, two-time Nobel Prize winner Linus Pauling and his followers recommend an intake somewhere between 2 to 9 grams a day during periods of health and even higher doses during times of stress or illness.[6,10,11] At the other end of the spectrum, the RDA has been established at 60 milligrams for adults.[3] While I lean toward Pauling's recommendation, I want to stress that you should not rely on supplements to meet all your vitamin C requirements. Vitamin C-rich foods are rich in compounds like flavonoids and carotenes which work to enhance the effects of vitamin C, as well as exert favorable effects of their own.

While most people think of citrus fruits as the best source of vitamin C, vegetables also contain high levels, especially broccoli, peppers, potatoes, and Brussels sprouts. Vitamin C is destroyed by exposure to air. So eat fresh foods as soon as possible after they come from the garden. Although a salad from a salad bar is a healthier lunch choice than a pastrami sandwich, the vitamin C content of the fruits and vegetables is only a fraction of what they would be if the salad were made fresh. For example, freshly sliced cucumbers, if left standing, will lose between 41% and 49% of their vitamin C content within the first 3 hours. A cantaloupe sliced, and left uncovered in the refrigerator, will lose 35% of its vitamin C content in less than 24 hours. My recommendation to individuals suffering from chronic fatigue (especially CFS) is that you eat foods rich in vitamin C and take an additional 500 to 9,000 milligrams of vitamin C daily. Take this amount in divided doses (usually three) rather than all at once. You will be able to determine how much vitamin C you need based on your gastrointestinal reaction. If you take too much vitamin C, it will usually cause much flatulence (gas) or watery diarrhea. Take an amount slightly below the level that causes these symptoms. This practice is referred to as taking vitamin C to bowel tolerance.

Magnesium

An extremely important mineral to sufferers of chronic fatigue, magnesium is the second most predominate mineral within our cells, next to potassium. Approximately 60% of the magnesium in the body is found in bone, 26% in muscle, and the remainder in soft tissue and body fluids. Magnesium's primary function is its ability to activate enzymes. Like potassium and other electrolytes, magnesium is involved in maintaining the electrical charge of cells, particularly muscles and nerves. Magnesium is involved in many cellular functions including energy production, protein formation, and cellular replication.[5]

Severe magnesium deficiency is characterized by mental confusion, irritability, weakness, heart disturbance, and problems in nerve conduction and muscle contraction. Other symptoms of magnesium deficiency may include muscle cramps, loss of appetite, insomnia, and a predisposition to stress.[5]

Magnesium deficiency is extremely common in the geriatric population and in women during the premenstrual period. Magnesium deficiency is often secondary to factors which reduce absorption or increase secretion such as high calcium intake, alcohol, surgery, diuretics, liver disease, kidney disease, and oral contraceptive use. The RDA for magnesium is 350 milligrams per day for adult males and 300 milligrams per day for adult females. For pregnant and lactating women the recommended allowance is 450 milligrams per day. Nutritional experts think that the ideal magnesium intake should be based on body weight (6 milligrams/kilograms body weight). For a 110-pound person, the recommendation would be 300 milligrams; for a 154-pound person, 420 milligrams; for a 200-pound person, 540 milligrams.

The average intake of magnesium by healthy adults in the United States ranges between 143 and 266 milligrams per day.[12] This is far below the RDA. Poor food choices are the main reason. Since magnesium occurs abundantly in whole foods, most nutritionists and dietitians assume that we get enough magnesium in our diet. But most Americans are not eating whole, natural foods. They are consuming large quantities of processed foods. Since food processing refines out a very large portion of magnesium, most Americans are not getting enough. What is the result of this low dietary magnesium? A higher susceptibility to a variety of diseases, including heart disease, high blood pressure, kidney stones, cancer, insomnia, PMS, and menstrual cramps.

The best dietary sources of magnesium are tofu, legumes, seeds, nuts, whole grains, and green leafy vegetables. Fish, meat, milk, and most commonly eaten fruits are quite low in magnesium. Most Americans consume a low magnesium diet because their diet is high in refined foods, meat, and dairy products.

Magnesium and Chronic Fatigue   An underlying magnesium deficiency, even if subclinical, can result in chronic fatigue and symptoms similar to CFS. Low red-blood-cell magnesium levels, a more accurate measure of magnesium status than routine blood analysis, have been found in many patients with chronic fatigue and CFS. This data alone suggests that magnesium supplementation may help improve energy levels.

Recently, researchers in the United Kingdom conducted a double-blind, placebo-controlled trial to assess the effect of magnesium supplementation on CFS.[13] Thirty-two patients received either an intramuscular injection of magnesium sulfate (1 gram in 2 milliliters injectable water) or a placebo (2 milliliters injectable water) for six weeks. At the end of the study, 12 of the 15 patients receiving magnesium reported significantly improved energy levels, better emotional states, and less pain, based on strict criteria. In contrast, only 3 of 17 placebo patients reported that they felt better and only 1 reported improved energy levels.

This study seems to confirm the impressive results obtained in clinical trials during the 1960s on patients suffering from chronic fatigue.[14-17] These studies utilized oral magnesium and potassium aspartate (1 gram each) rather than injectable magnesium. Between 75% and 91% of the nearly 3,000 patients studied experienced relief of fatigue during treatment with the magnesium and potassium aspartate. In contrast, the number of patients responding to the placebo was between 9% and 26%. The beneficial effect was usually noted after only four to five days, but sometimes ten days were required. Patients usually continued treatment for four to six weeks; afterwards, in many cases fatigue did not return.

Injectable magnesium is not necessary to restore magnesium status.[18] Absorption studies indicate that magnesium is easily absorbed orally when it is bound to aspartate or citrate. Both of these compounds may also help fight off fatigue. Aspartate feeds into the Krebs cycle, the final common pathway for the conversion of glucose, fatty acids, and amino acids to chemical energy (ATP), while citrate is itself a component of Krebs cycle. Krebs cycle components (including aspartate, citrate, fumarate, malate, and succinate) usually provide a better mineral chelate; evidence suggests that minerals chelated to the Krebs cycle intermediates are better absorbed, utilized, and tolerated compared to inorganic or relatively insoluble mineral salts including magnesium chloride, oxide, or carbonate.[18,19]

Components of the Krebs cycle are able to bind two or three mineral molecules for every one of its own molecules. The Krebs cycle mineral chelates also have effervescent qualities which ionize the minerals, thereby greatly increasing bioavailability. In addition, the intermediates have some properties of their own that suggest further benefits, such as their ability to chelate out heavy metals and decrease fatigue.

Several major suppliers of nutritional products offer magnesium bound to the Krebs cycle intermediates. I recommend that you use this form. If you cannot locate Krebs cycle chelates at your health food store, look for either magnesium aspartate or citrate. Take an additional 250 to 400 milligrams of magnesium from this source in addition to your multiple vitamin-mineral to achieve a total daily intake of 500 to 750 milligrams of magnesium from your supplements.

In my clinical practice, in most instances, I prefer using a balanced mineral formula rather than isolated mineral chelates. When any single mineral is taken at high dosages it can impair the absorption of other important minerals. For example, I usually use a multiple mineral formula (Krebs Cycle Chelates from Enzymatic Therapy) to achieve the proper levels of magnesium. Many other manufacturers of nutritional supplements provide multi-mineral formulas featuring the Krebs cycle intermediates.

Iron

Iron deficiency is a frequent cause of chronic fatigue. A severe deficiency of iron is the most common cause of anemia, a condition in which the blood is deficient in red blood cells or the hemoglobin (iron-containing) portion of red blood cells. The symptoms of anemia, including extreme fatigue as well as cold hands and feet, reflect a lack of oxygen being delivered to tissues and a build-up of carbon dioxide. The symptoms reflect iron's central role in the hemoglobin molecule of our red blood cells. The red blood cells, with the help of hemoglobin, function in transporting oxygen from the lungs to the body's tissues and the transportation of carbon dioxide from the tissues to the lungs.

It must be pointed out that anemia is the last stage of iron deficiency. Several researchers have clearly demonstrated that even slight iron-deficiency anemia leads to fatigue and a reduction in physical work capacity and productivity.[20,21] Impaired physical performance due to iron deficiency is not dependent on anemia.[22] The iron-dependent enzymes involved in energy production and metabolism will be impaired long before anemia occurs.

Relying on routine blood analysis for the diagnosis of iron deficiency is not accurate enough. Serum ferritin is the best laboratory test for determining body iron stores. I always include a serum ferritin determination in my routine analysis of women with chronic fatigue. In men, I may suspect iron deficiency may be playing a role if they have a history of peptic ulcers, hemorrhoids, blood loss, or long-term use of antacids.

Dietary Sources of Iron   There are two forms of dietary iron, "heme" iron and "non-heme" iron. Heme iron is iron bound to hemoglobin and myoglobin, and is found in liver and other meats. It is the most efficiently absorbed form of iron, with an approximate absorption rate of 25%. Non-heme iron is found in plant foods and most iron supplements. Non-heme iron has an approximate absorption rate of 5%.[23]

Heme iron is absorbed intact while non-heme iron is dependent upon ionization by stomach acid and complex transport mechanisms. In addition, non-heme iron is extremely susceptible to blocking agents such as fiber, phosphates, calcium, tannates, and preservatives, while heme iron is not affected by these factors. Non-heme iron also requires the presence of stomach acid. Lack of stomach acid makes it difficult for many people to absorb iron.[24,25]

Iron Supplements   Iron supplementation is often required to build up iron levels. Beef (bovine) liver extracts provide the best form of iron—heme iron—and are, therefore, considered the best iron supplements. Liver extracts not only contain iron, but also other nutritional and physiological substances which promote healthy red blood cells. Many commercially available liver extracts provide the benefit of heme iron without the calories and fat that would be required to achieve similar amounts of heme iron from the dietary intake of liver and other meats. If you are iron-deficient take two 500-milligram tablets or capsules of liver extract with your meals.

Despite the superiority of heme iron, non-heme iron salts are the most popular iron supplements. One reason is that even though heme iron is better absorbed, it is easy to take higher quantities of non-heme iron salts so that the net amount of iron absorbed is about equal. In other words, if you take 3 milligrams of heme iron and 50 milligrams of non-heme iron, the net absorption for each will be about the same.

If you are iron-deficient and want to take a non-heme source, take 30 milligrams of iron bound to either succinate or fumarate twice daily between meals. If this recommendation results in abdominal discomfort, take 30 milligrams with meals three times daily.

In my clinical practice, when serum ferritin values are low, I tend to recommend a formula containing both heme and non-heme iron. Each capsule contains 30 milligrams of ferrous succinate along with 250 milligrams of liver fractions, a rich source of heme iron. In addition, other blood-building factors including vitamin C, folic acid, vitamin B12, and fat-soluble chlorophyll are provided. If you want to use this formula (Ultimate Iron from Enzymatic Therapy), take 1 capsule twice daily between meals or 1 capsule with meals three times daily.

Other Benefits of Liver   In men and women with normal serum ferritin values who suffer from chronic fatigue, I will often recommend liver extracts, not so much for the heme iron content, but rather for the endurance-enhancing effects of liver. In the 1950s, Dr. B. H. Ershoff of the University of Southern California performed several experiments that demonstrated that raw liver has phenomenal anti-fatigue effects. In one of Dr. Ershoff's classic experiments, three groups of laboratory rats were fed different diets over a twelve-week period. The first group was fed a usual laboratory diet to which 11 different vitamins were added. The second group was fed the same diet plus all known B vitamins. The third group was fed the original diet with 10% raw liver in place of the vitamins.

At the end of the 12 weeks each group of rats was placed in drums of water which they could not climb out of. The first group of rats swam for an average of 13.3 minutes, the second group averaged 13.4 minutes before giving up, indicating that all available strength and energy had been exhausted. The third group, however, demonstrated amazing results. Three rats swam for 63, 83, and 87 minutes, while the balance of the group were still swimming vigorously at the end of the 2-hour test period.

The mysterious effects of liver have puzzled researchers and scientists for decades. Liver seems to contain a physiological substance that has not yet been identified which promotes stamina, strength, and endurance. These attributes have made liver preparations extremely popular among bodybuilders and athletes.

Liver Extracts to Enhance Liver Function   Liver extracts have long been used to improve liver function. In fact, they have been used in the treatment of many chronic liver diseases since 1896. Numerous scientific investigations into the therapeutic efficacy of liver extracts have demonstrated that these extracts possess an ability to improve fat utilization, promote tissue regeneration, and prevent damage to the liver.[26-29] In short, clinical studies have demonstrated that oral administration of liver extracts can be quite effective in improving liver function.

For example, in one double-blind study involving 556 patients with chronic hepatitis the patients were given either 70 milligrams of liver hydrosylate or a placebo three times daily.[29] At the end of three months of treatment, the group receiving the liver extract was shown to have far lower liver enzyme levels. Since the level of liver enzymes in the blood reflect damage to the liver, it can be concluded that the liver extract is effective in chronic hepatitis due to its ability to repair damaged liver cells as well as prevent further damage to the liver.

Since the liver is the most important organ of metabolism, when liver function improves, metabolism improves. An improved metabolism creates high energy levels and greater feelings of health and well-being.

Choosing a High-Quality Liver Extract
he best liver products are usually made from beef liver obtained from animals raised in South America, where ranchers use no chemical sprays, pesticides, or antibiotics in their livestock feed.

Most clinical studies have utilized hydrolyzed liver extracts produced by exposing the liver material to enzymes which hydrolyze (add water to) the protein bonds. This process basically "liquifies" the liver and is the reason why hydrolyzed extracts are often referred to as "liquid liver extracts." If you see a product labeled Liquid Liver, don't worry, you will not have to swallow a liquid. Suppliers provide the liquid liver in capsule form.

In my clinical practice, I tend to use a product called Liquid Liver Extract with Siberian Ginseng from Enzymatic Therapy which combines a specific hydrolyzed liver fraction (550 milligrams per capsule) and a very concentrated Siberian ginseng extract (25 milligrams per capsule). My usual recommendation is two capsules three times daily until energy levels are restored. Once energy levels are restored, I will have the patient reduce the dose gradually (reduce daily dosage by one capsule every week).

Chapter Summary

In the treatment of chronic fatigue, nutritional supplementation is often essential. A deficiency of virtually any nutrient can produce symptoms of fatigue as well as render the body susceptible to infection.

In an effort to establish optimum nutritional status, in addition to the dietary recommendations given in Chapter 4, individuals with chronic fatigue should follow the guidelines for nutritional supplementation outlined in this chapter. These guidelines can best be met by taking a high-potency multiple vitamin-mineral formula, along with extra vitamin C and minerals (especially magnesium).

A special nutritional supplement that is often quite useful in re-establishing energy levels is hydrolyzed (liquid) liver extract. These liver preparations are rich in many nutrients including heme iron and vitamin B12. In addition, the stamina- and endurance-enhancing effects of liver are well known.

Addressing the Causes of Chronic Fatigue

7

Chronic Fatigue and Liver Function

To a very large extent your health, vitality, and energy levels are determined by the health and vitality of your liver. The liver is truly an intricate, complex, and remarkable organ. It is, without question, the most important organ of metabolism.

The liver deals with a constant onslaught of toxic chemicals from the body and its environment. Toxic chemicals are everywhere—in the air we breathe and the water and food we consume. Some of the toxic chemicals known to pass through the liver include: heavy metals like lead, cadmium, mercury, and aluminum; solvents like formaldehyde, toluene, and acetone; the polycyclic hydrocarbons that are components of various herbicides and pesticides, including DDT, dioxin, 2,4,5-T, 2,4-D; and the halogenated compounds PCB and PCP. Although the exact degree to which Americans are exposed to these compounds is not known, it is probably quite high, as yearly production of synthetic organic pesticides alone exceeds 1.4 billion pounds and the United States is known to dump over 600,000 tons of lead into the atmosphere each year.[1,2]

It is quite possible that the increasing number of people with chronic fatigue may be a result of increased pollution. Although the full health effects of chronic exposure to toxic compounds has not been determined, they are known to be linked to many symptoms common to individuals with chronic fatigue (see Chapter 2). My experience is that every patient with chronic fatigue can benefit from liver-supportive therapy as detailed in this chapter.

The Liver and Immune Function

The health and function of the liver is critically linked to the status of the immune system. Although not technically considered an organ of the immune system or a lymphatic organ, the liver plays a role in a variety of functions essential to a healthy immune system. Specifically, the liver produces several physiological substances required by the immune system; is the major producer of lymph in the body; and with the help of special white blood cells known as Kupffer cells, is responsible for filtering the blood and removing cellular debris, bacteria, viruses, yeast, and toxic foreign compounds that would otherwise be absorbed by the gastrointestinal tract. Kupffer cells, when functioning properly, have been shown to engulf and destroy a single bacteria in less than one one-hundredth of a second.

Damage to the Liver and Chronic Fatigue

Damage to the liver is often an underlying factor in chronic fatigue, including CFS. When the liver is even slightly damaged by chemical toxins, immune function is severely compromised.

The immunosuppressive effect of nonviral liver damage has been repeatedly demonstrated in experimental animal studies and human studies. For example, when the liver of a rat is damaged by a chemical toxin, its immune function is severely hindered.[3] Liver injury is also linked to candida overgrowth, as evident in studies in mice demonstrating that when the liver is even slightly damaged, candida run rampant through the body.[4]

The classic human example of the effect of liver injury on immune function is seen with excess alcohol consumption. This is most evident in the alcoholic, but in some individuals ingestion of as little as one to two ounces of alcohol is enough to induce sufficient injury and lead to immune suppression. The levels of antioxidant nutrients like vitamin C, vitamin E, selenium, and zinc appear to be the critical factors which determine the extent of immune system impairment after alcohol ingestion.

Antioxidants are essential in protecting the liver from damage. Optimum tissue concentrations of these compounds should be maintained in the treatment of hepatic disease as well as in the promotion of liver health.

Supporting the Liver

A rational approach to aiding the body's detoxification involves: (1) eating a diet which focuses on fresh fruits and vegetables, whole grains, legumes, nuts, and seeds; (2) adopting a healthy lifestyle including avoiding alcohol and exercising regularly; (3) taking a high-potency multiple vitamin and mineral supplement; (4) using special nutritional and herbal supplements to protect the liver and enhance liver function; and (5) going on a 3-day fast at the change of each season.

Diet and Liver Function

The first step in supporting proper liver function is to follow the dietary recommendations given in Chapter 4. Such a diet will provide the liver with the wide range of essential nutri-ents it needs to carry on its important functions. If you want to have a healthy liver, there are three things you definitely want to stay away from: (1) saturated fats; (2) refined sugar; and (3) alcohol. A diet high in saturated fats increases the risk of developing fatty infiltration and/or cholestasis (see Chapter 2). In contrast, a diet rich in dietary fiber, particularly the water-soluble fibers, has a choleretic effect by promoting increased bile secretion.

Special foods rich in factors which help protect the liver from damage and improve liver function include: high sulfur-containing foods like garlic, legumes, onions, and eggs; good sources of water-soluble fibers such as pears, oat bran, apples, and legumes; cabbage-family vegetables, especially broccoli, Brussels sprouts, and cabbage; and artichokes, beets, carrots, dandelion, and many herbs and spices like turmeric, cinnamon, and licorice.

Alcohol and the Liver   Alcohol inhibits detoxification processes and can lead to liver damage and immune sup-pression. If you suffer from chronic fatigue, I recommend that you eliminate alcohol entirely. After you have regained your vigor, if you are going to drink, limit yourself to one drink and be sure to employ all the other measures to support the liver.

High-Potency Multiple Vitamin and Mineral Formulas
In trying to deal with all the toxic chemicals we are constant-ly exposed to, antioxidant vitamins like vitamin C, beta-carotene, and vitamin E are obviously quite important in protecting the liver from damage as well as helping in detoxification mechanisms, but even simple nutrients like B vitamins, calcium, and trace minerals are critical in the elimination of heavy metals and other toxic compounds from the body.[5–7] Taking a high-potency multiple vitamin and min-eral is a must.

Special Nutritional Factors

The use of liver extracts to enhance liver function was discussed in Chapter 6. In addition, choline, betaine, and methionine are often beneficial. These nutrients are referred to as "lipotropic agents," compounds which promote the flow of fat and bile to and from the liver. In essence, they produce a "decongestant" effect on the liver and promote improved liver function and fat metabolism.

Formulas containing lipotropic agents are very useful in enhancing detoxification reactions and other liver functions. Lipotropic formulas have been used for a wide variety of conditions by nutrition-oriented physicians including a number of liver disorders including hepatitis, cirrhosis, and chemical-induced liver disease.

Most major manufacturers of nutritional supplements offer lipotropic formulas. The important thing, when taking a lipotropic formula, is to take enough of the formula to provide a daily dose of 1,000 milligrams of choline and 1,000 milligrams of either methionine or cysteine.

Lipotropic formulas appear to increase the levels of two important liver substances: SAM (S-adenosylmethionine), the major lipotropic compound in the liver, and glutathione, one of the liver's major detoxifying compounds.[8,9]

SAM (S-adenosylmethionine) SAM is made in the liver from the essential amino acid methionine. SAM is available in Europe as a drug and has been shown to be quite beneficial in restoring liver function.[8–10] Although it is not currently available in the United States, various lipotropic factors, including methionine, choline, and betaine, have been shown to increase the natural levels of SAM in the liver.[11–13]

Glutathione The levels of methionine consumed in the diet is a major determinate of the level of SAM and glutathione.

Glutathione is a peptide (small protein) composed of three amino acids: cysteine (can be formed from methionine), glutamic acid, and glycine. Glutathione assumes a critical role in defense against a variety of injurious agents by combining directly with toxic substances to neutralize them.

Many toxic chemicals, including heavy metals, are fat-soluble. This makes it very difficult for the body to eliminate them. The only way the body can effectively eliminate fat-soluble compounds is by excreting them in the bile. The problem is that 99% of the bile, including the excreted toxins, is reabsorbed. Fortunately, the body is able to convert the fat-soluble toxins into a water-soluble form. The body performs this feat with the help of glutathione. When glutathione binds to a fat-soluble toxin it ultimately converts it to a water-soluble form, allowing more efficient excretion via the kidneys. The elimination of heavy metals, like mercury and lead, is dependent upon adequate levels of glutathione, which in turn is dependent upon adequate levels of methionine and cysteine.[14-16]

When increased levels of toxic compounds are present, more methionine is converted to cysteine and glutathione synthesis. Methionine and cysteine have a protective effect on glutathione and prevent depletion during toxic overload.[17] This helps protect the liver from the damaging effects of toxic compounds and promotes their elimination.

Plant-Based Medicines and Liver Function

A long list of plants are known to exert beneficial effects on liver function. The most impressive research has been done on a special extract of milk thistle (*Silybum marianum*) known as silymarin. Silymarin refers to a group of flavonoid compounds which have been shown to have a tremendous effect on protecting the liver from damage as well as enhancing the body's detoxification processes.

Silymarin prevents damage to the liver by acting as an antioxidant.[18-20] Silymarin is many times more potent in antioxidant activity than vitamin E and vitamin C.[18]

The protective effect of silymarin against liver damage has been demonstrated in a number of experimental studies. Experimental liver damage in animals is produced by extremely toxic chemicals such as carbon tetrachloride, amanita toxin, galactosamine, and praseodymium nitrate. Silymarin has been shown to protect against liver damage by all of these agents.[18-20]

Silymarin enhances detoxification reaction mainly by preventing the depletion of glutathione. As discussed above, the level of glutathione in the liver is critically linked to the liver's ability to detoxify. The higher the glutathione content, the greater the liver's capacity to detoxify harmful chemicals. Typically, when we are exposed to chemicals which can damage the liver (including alcohol), the concentration of glutathione in the liver is substantially reduced. This reduction in glutathione makes the liver cells susceptible to damage. Silymarin not only prevents the depletion of glutathione induced by alcohol and other toxic chemicals, but has been shown to increase the level of glutathione of the liver by up to 35%.[21] Since the ability of the liver to detoxify is largely related to the level of glutathione in the liver, the results of this study seem to indicate that silymarin can increase detoxification reactions by up to 35%.

In human studies, silymarin has been shown to have positive effects in treating liver diseases of various kinds, including cirrhosis, chronic hepatitis, fatty infiltration of the liver (chemical- and alcohol-induced fatty liver), and inflammation of the bile duct.[22-26]

Silymarin products are available at health food stores. The standard dosage for silymarin is 70–210 milligrams three times daily.

Fasting

Often used as a detoxification method, fasting is one of the quickest ways to increase elimination of wastes and enhance the healing processes of the body. Fasting is defined as abstinence from all food and drink except water for a specific period of time, usually for a therapeutic or religious purpose.

Although therapeutic fasting is probably one of the oldest known therapies it has been largely ignored by the medical community, despite the fact that significant scientific research on fasting exists in the medical literature. Numerous medical journals have carried articles on the use of fasting in the treatment of obesity, chemical poisoning, rheumatoid arthritis, allergies, psoriasis, eczema, thrombophlebitis, leg ulcers, irritable bowel syndrome, impaired or deranged appetite, bronchial asthma, depression, neurosis, and schizophrenia.

A significant study on fasting and detoxification appeared in the *American Journal of Industrial Medicine* in 1984.[27] This study involved patients who had ingested rice oil contaminated with polychlorinated biphenyls (PCBs). All patients reported improvement in symptoms, and some observed "dramatic" relief, after undergoing 7- to 10-day fasts. This research supports past studies of PCB-poisoned patients and indicates the therapeutic effects of fasting as an aid to detoxification.

It is important to point out that caution must be used when fasting. Please consult a physician before going on any unsupervised fast.

If you elect to try a fast, it is a good idea to support detoxification reactions, especially if you are particularly toxic or have a long history of exposure to fat-soluble toxins like pesticides. The reason is that during a fast, stored toxins in our fat cells are released into the system. For example, the pesticide DDT has been shown to be mobilized during a fast and may reach blood levels toxic to the nervous system.[6]

One of the best ways to support detoxification reactions during a fast is to go on a 3-day fresh juice fast rather than a water fast or a longer fast. Longer fasts require strict medical supervision, preferably at an in-patient facility, but a short fast can usually be conducted at home. Before starting any unsupervised fast, however, it is a very good idea to consult your physician.

A 3-day juice fast consists of three or four 8- to 12- ounce juice meals spread throughout the day. During this period your body will begin ridding stored toxins. Drinking fresh juice for cleansing reduces some of the side effects associated with a water fast such as light-headedness, tiredness, or headaches. While on a fresh juice fast, individuals typically experience an increased sense of well-being, renewed energy, clearer thought, and a sense of purity.

To further aid in detoxification, use the following guidelines:

1. Take a high-potency multiple vitamin and mineral formula to provide general support.
2. Take a lipotropic formula according to the guidelines on page 121.
3. Take 1,000 milligrams of vitamin C three times daily.
4. Take 1 to 2 tablespoons of a fiber supplement at night before retiring. The best fiber sources are the water-soluble fibers such as powdered psyllium seed husks, guar gum, and oat bran.
5. If you are particularly toxic, take silymarin at a dosage of 70 to 210 milligrams three times daily.

Tips on Fasting

- Although a short juice fast can be started at any time, it is best to begin on a weekend or during a time period when adequate rest can be assured. The more rest you can get, the better the results as your energy can be directed toward healing instead of supporting other body functions.

- Prepare for a fast on the day before solid food is stopped by making the last meal consist only of fresh fruits and vegetables (some authorities recommend a full day of raw food to start a fast, even a juice fast).

- Consume only fresh fruit and vegetable juices (ideally prepared from organic produce) for 3 to 5 days. Drink four 8- to 12-ounce glasses of fresh juice throughout the day. In addition to the fresh juice, drink pure water according to your thirst, at least four 8-ounce glasses every day of the fast.

- Do not drink coffee, bottled, canned, or frozen juice, or soft drinks. Herbal teas can be quite supportive of a fast, but they should not be sweetened.

- Exercise is not usually encouraged while fasting. It is a good idea to conserve energy and allow maximal healing. Short walks or light stretching are useful, but heavy workouts tax the system and inhibit repair and elimination.

- Rest is one of the most important aspects of a fast. A nap or two during the day is recommended. Less sleep will usually be required at night, since daily activity is lower. Body temperature usually drops during a fast, as does blood pressure, and pulse and respiratory rate—all measures of the slowing of the metabolic rate of the body. It is important, therefore, to stay warm.

- When it is time to break your fast, reintroduce solid foods gradually by limiting portions. Do not overeat. Eat slowly, chew thoroughly, and eat foods at room temperature.

Chapter Summary

Detoxification of harmful substances is a continual process in the body. The body's ability to eliminate toxins largely determines an individual's health status, including the health of the immune system. A number of toxins such as heavy metals, solvents, pesticides, and microbial toxins are known to cause significant health problems and are thought to play a major role in some individuals with chronic fatigue.

A rational approach to aiding the body's detoxification mechanisms involves adopting a healthy diet and lifestyle and using nutritional and herbal products which protect and support the functions of the liver. A 3-day juice fast at the change of seasons is also a good way to help prevent the accumulation of toxic substances in the body.

8

Chronic Fatigue and Immune Function

Recurrent or chronic infections, including CFS and chronic candidiasis, are characterized by a depressed immune system. What makes it difficult to overcome such illness is a repetitive cycle: a compromised immune system leads to infection, and infection damages the immune system, further weakening resistance. Enhancing the immune system by following the guidelines in this chapter may provide an answer to chronic fatigue. Restoring healthy immune function is especially important in the case of CFS.

Too often in conventional medicine a patient's relative susceptibility to infection or disease is overlooked. Support and enhancement of immune system function (including enhancing the function of the liver) is perhaps the most vital step in achieving host resistance and reducing susceptibility.

What Is the Immune System?

One of the most complex and fascinating systems of the human body, the immune system's prime function is to protect the body against infection and the development of cancer.

The immune system is composed of the lymphatic vessels and organs (thymus, spleen, tonsils, and lymph nodes), white blood cells (lymphocytes, neutrophils, basophils, eosinophils, monocytes, etc.), specialized cells residing in various tissue (macrophages, mast cells, etc.), and specialized serum factors.

The Thymus

The thymus is the major gland of our immune system. It is composed of two soft pinkish-gray lobes lying in a bib-like fashion just below the thyroid gland and above the heart. To a very large extent, the health of the thymus determines the health of the immune system. Individuals who get frequent infections or suffer from chronic infections typically have impaired thymus activity. Also, people afflicted with hayfever, allergies, migraine headaches, or rheumatoid arthritis usually have an altered thymus function.

The thymus is responsible for many immune system functions including the production of T lymphocytes, a type of white blood cell responsible for "cell-mediated immunity." Cell-mediated immunity refers to immune mechanisms not controlled or mediated by antibodies.

Cell-mediated immunity is critical in the resistance to infection by mold-like bacteria, yeast (including Candida albicans), fungi, parasites, and viruses (including Herpes simplex, Epstein–Barr, and viruses that cause hepatitis). If an individual is suffering from an infection from these organisms it is a good indication that their cell-mediated immunity is not functioning up to par. Cell-mediated immunity also helps protect against the development of cancer, auto-immune disorders like rheumatoid arthritis, and allergies.

The thymus gland releases several hormones such as thymosin, thymopoeitin, and serum thymic factor which regulate many immune functions. Low levels of these hormones in the blood are associated with depressed immunity and an increased susceptibility to infection. Typically, thymic hormone levels will be very low in the elderly, individuals prone to infection, and cancer and AIDS patients, and when an individual is exposed to undue stress.

Lymph, Lymphatic Vessels, and Lymph Nodes

Approximately one-sixth of the entire body consists of the space between cells. Collectively, this space is referred to as the interstitium, and the fluid contained within the space is referred to as the interstitial fluid. This fluid flows into the lymphatic vessels and becomes the lymph.

Lymphatic vessels usually run parallel to arteries and veins. These vessels drain waste products from tissues and transport lymph to the lymph nodes, which function in filtering the lymph. The cells responsible for filtering the lymph are macrophages. These large cells engulf and destroy foreign particles, including bacteria and cellular debris.

The lymph nodes also contain B-lymphocytes, the white blood cells which are capable of initiating antibody production in response to the presence of viruses, bacteria, yeast, and other unwanted organisms.

The Spleen

The spleen is the largest mass of lymphatic tissue in the body. Weighing about 7 ounces, the spleen is a fist-sized, spongy, dark purple organ that lies in the upper left abdomen behind the lower ribs. The spleen's functions include producing white blood cells, engulfing and destroying bacteria and cellular debris, and destroying worn-out red blood cells and platelets. The spleen also serves as a blood-reservoir. During times of high demand, such as hemorrhage, the spleen can release its stored blood and prevent shock.

Like the thymus, the spleen releases many potent immune system-enhancing compounds. For example, tuftsin and splenopentin, two small peptides secreted by the spleen, as well as spleen extracts, have been shown to exert profound immune-enhancing activity.[1-4]

White Blood Cells

There are several types of white blood cells, including neutrophils, eosinophils, basophils, lymphocytes, and monocytes.

Neutrophils   These cells actively phagocytize—engulf and destroy—bacteria, tumor cells, and dead particulate matter. Neutrophils are especially important in preventing bacterial infection.

Eosinophils and Basophils   These cells are involved in allergic conditions. They secrete histamine and other compounds designed to break down antigen-antibody complexes. They also promote allergic mechanisms.

Lymphocytes   There are several types of lymphocytes including T cells, B cells, and natural killer cells.

T cells

T cells stand for thymus derived lymphocytes. These cells orchestrate many immune functions and are the major components of cell-mediated immunity (discussed above). There are different types of T cells including helper T cells which help other white blood cells to function; suppressor T cells which inhibit white blood cell functions; and cytotoxic T cells which attack and destroy foreign tissue, cancer cells, and virus infected cells.

T-Cell Ratios

The ratio of helper T cells to suppressor T cells is a useful determinant of immune function. If the ratio is low, immunodeficiency is present. For example, AIDS is characterized by a very low ratio. If the ratio of helper T cells to suppressor T cells is high, allergies or autoimmune disorders like rheumatoid arthritis and lupus are usually present. Both high and low T-cell ratios have been found in CFS.

B Cells

B cells are responsible for producing antibodies—large protein molecules which bind to foreign molecules (antigens) on bacteria, viruses, other organisms, and tumor cells. After the antibody binds to the antigen it sets up a sequence of events that ultimately destroys the infectious organism or tumor cell.

Natural Killer Cells

As mentioned in Chapter 1, natural killer cells (or NK cells) received their name because of their ability to destroy cells that have become cancerous or infected with viruses. They are the body's first line of defense against cancer development. The level or activity of natural killer cells in CFS is usually low.

Monocytes   Monocytes are the garbage collectors of the body. These large white blood cells are responsible for cleaning up cellular debris after an infection. Monocytes are also responsible for triggering many immune responses.

Special Tissue Cells

Macrophages   As stated earlier, lymph is filtered by specialized cells known as macrophages. Macrophages are actually monocytes that have taken up residence in specific tissues like the liver, spleen, and lymph nodes. These large cells phagocytize (engulf) foreign particles including bacteria and cellular debris. Macrophages are essential in protecting against invasion by microorganisms and damage to the lymphatic system.

Mast Cells   Mast cells are basophils which have taken up residence primarily along blood vessels. The mast cell, like the basophil, is responsible for releasing histamine and other compounds involved in allergic reactions.

Special Chemical Factors

A number of special chemical factors enhance the immune system: interferon, interleukin II, and complement fractions. These compounds are produced by various white blood cells, for example, interferon is produced primarily by T cells, interleukins are produced by macrophages and T cells, and complement fractions are manufactured in the liver and spleen. These special chemical factors are extremely important in activating the white blood cells to destroy cancer cells and viruses.

Supporting the Immune System

In the individual with CFS, supporting the immune system is critical to re-establishing energy levels and vitality. There really isn't any single magic bullet which can immediately restore healthy immune function. Instead, a comprehensive approach involving lifestyle, stress management, exercise, diet, nutritional supplementation, glandular therapy, and the use of plant-based medicines is used.

Influence of Mood and Attitude

Our mood and attitude has a tremendous bearing on the function of our immune system. When we are happy and up, our immune system functions much better. Conversely, when we are depressed, our immune system tends to be depressed. Employing the measures outlined in Chapter 3 can be quite useful in improving the health of the immune system.

Influence of Stress

Stress causes the adrenal gland hormones, including adrenaline and corticosteroids, to increase. Among other things, these hormones inhibit white blood cells and cause the thymus gland to shrink (involute). This leads to a significant suppression of immune function, leaving the host susceptible to infections, cancer, and other illnesses. The level of immune suppression is usually proportional to the level of stress.

Stress results in stimulation of the sympathetic nervous system which is responsible for the fight or flight response. The immune system functions better under parasympathetic nervous system tone. This portion of our autonomic nervous system assumes control over bodily functions during periods of rest, relaxation, visualization, meditation, and sleep. During the deepest levels of sleep, potent immune-enhancing compounds are released and many immune functions are greatly increased.[5] The value of good deep sleep and relaxation techniques for counteracting the effects of stress and enhancing our immune system cannot be overemphasized.

Influence of Lifestyle

A healthy lifestyle goes a long way in establishing a healthy immune system. Of particular interest to individuals with CFS are the results of several studies which have examined the effect of lifestyle on natural killer cell activity.[6,7] As noted in Chapter 1, reduced natural killer cell number or activity is one of the hallmark features of CFS. The following practices are associated with higher natural killer cell activity:

1. Not smoking
2. Increased intake of green vegetables
3. Regular meals
4. Proper body weight
5. More than 7 hours of sleep
6. Regular exercise
7. A vegetarian diet

Diet and Immune Function

The health of the immune system gland is largely determined by your state of stress and nutritional status. Dietary factors which depress immune function include nutrient deficiency, sugar, and high cholesterol levels in the blood. Dietary factors which enhance immune function include all essential nutrients, antioxidants, carotenes, and flavonoids.

Consistent with good health, optimal immune function requires a healthy diet that is (1) rich in whole, natural foods, such as fruits, vegetables, grains, beans, seeds, and nuts, (2) low in fats and refined sugars, and (3) contains adequate, but not excessive, amounts of protein. On top of this, for optimum immune function, an individual should consume 16 to 24 ounces of fresh fruit or vegetable juice per day, and drink five or six 8-ounce glasses of water per day (preferably pure). These dietary recommendations, along with a positive mental attitude, a good high-potency multiple vitamin-mineral supplement, a regular exercise program of at least 30 minutes of aerobic exercise, daily deep breathing and relaxation exercises such as meditation or prayer, and at least 7 hours of sleep daily will go a long way in helping the immune system function at an optimum level.

Let's take a closer look at some of the specific dietary factors which can play a role in immune function.

Nutrient Deficiency

Nutrient deficiency is the most frequent cause of a depressed immune system. In nutrition surveys it has been shown that most Americans are deficient in at least one nutrient. Several studies have estimated that 19% to 66% of the elderly population consume two-thirds or less of the RDA for various nutrients.[8] The significance of these findings is substantial, as virtually any nutrient deficiency will result in an impaired immune system, increasing your risk for cancer and infections.

Obesity and Elevated Fats in the Blood

Americans are typically overfed, but undernourished. The nutritional deficiencies plus the excesses team up to greatly reduce immune function. Obesity is not only associated with such conditions as atherosclerosis, hypertension, diabetes mellitus, and joint disorders, it is also associated with decreased immune status, as evidenced by the decreased bacteria-killing activity of neutrophils, and increased morbidity and mortality from infections and cancer.[9]

Since cholesterol and fat levels in the blood are usually elevated in obese individuals, this may explain their impaired immune function. Increased blood levels of cholesterol, free fatty acids, triglycerides, and bile acids inhibit various immune functions.[9] Optimal immune function is therefore dependent on maintaining healthy levels of cholesterol and other fats in the blood.

Sugar

The high-sugar diet of many Americans may be contributing to a general state of immune suppression and increased susceptibility to infections. Ingestion of excess sugar has been definitively shown to adversely affect the immune system.[10-12] Considering that the average American consumes 150 grams of sucrose, plus other refined simple sugars, each day, the inescapable conclusion is that most Americans have chronically depressed immune systems. It is clear, particularly during an infection or chronic illness including CFS, that the consumption of refined sugars is harmful to immune function.

Thymus Gland Activity and Immune Function

Perhaps the most effective method in re-establishing a healthy immune system is employing measures designed to improve thymus function. Promoting optimal thymus gland activity involves: (1) prevention of thymic involution or shrinkage by ensuring adequate dietary intake of antioxidant nutrients like carotenes, vitamin C, vitamin E, zinc, and selenium; (2) the intake of specific nutrients required in the manufacture or action of thymic hormones; and (3) using products containing concentrates of calf thymus tissue.

Antioxidants and Thymus Function

The thymus gland shows maximum development immediately after birth. As we age the thymus gland undergoes a process of shrinkage or involution. The reason for this involution is that the thymus gland is extremely susceptible to free radical and oxidative damage caused by stress, radiation, infection, and chronic illness.

It is thought that individuals with CFS suffer from a state of oxidative imbalance. In other words, these patients have a greater number of pro-oxidants in their system than antioxidants. If this is true, antioxidant therapy holds great promise in the treatment of CFS.

Juicing fresh fruits and vegetables to increase intake of antioxidant compounds appears to be a wise recommendation in chronic fatigue patients. In addition, it is important to supplement the diet with antioxidants such as vitamin C, vitamin E, selenium, zinc, and beta-carotene. All of these nutrients have been shown to prevent thymic involution and enhance cell-mediated immune function.[13-16] Follow the recommendations given in Chapter 6.

In addition to boosting general immune function and protecting the thymus from damage, vitamin C has been shown to enhance natural killer cell activity—a critical goal in treating CFS. In one study, when 20 healthy subjects were given 60 milligrams of vitamin C per kilogram (2.2 pounds) of body weight, natural killer cell activity increased up to an incredible 231%.[17] The increase in activity continued steadily for the first 24 hours and returned to normal after 48 hours. It is unlikely that lower doses of vitamin C would be as effective in producing these effects. The results of this study provide further evidence for the need to take an additional 3 to 8 grams of vitamin C per day if you suffer from an impaired immune system.

Nutrients and Thymic Hormone Manufacture

Many nutrients function as significant cofactors in the manufacture, secretion, and function of thymic hormones. Deficiencies of any one of these nutrients results in decreased thymic hormone action and impaired immune function. Zinc, vitamin B6, and vitamin C are the most critical nutrients. Supplementation with these nutrients has been shown to increase thymic hormone function and cell-mediated immunity.[14,15] Following the guidelines in Chapter 6 will provide optimal levels of these important nutrients.

Zinc is perhaps the most critical nutrient involved in thymus gland function and thymus hormone action. Zinc is involved in virtually every aspect of immunity. When zinc levels are low, the number of T cells is reduced; thymic hormone levels are lower, and many white-blood-cell functions critical to the immune response are severely lacking. All of these effects are reversible with adequate zinc administration.[18,19]

Thymus Extracts and Thymus Function

A substantial amount of clinical data supports the effectiveness of orally administered calf thymus extracts in restoring and enhancing immune function.[20,21] The effectiveness of thymus extract is reflective of broad spectrum immune system enhancement, presumably mediated by improved thymus gland activity. This effect fits in nicely with one of the basic concepts of glandular therapy, that is, that the oral ingestion of glandular material of a certain animal gland will strengthen the corresponding human gland. The result is a broad general effect indicative of improved glandular function.

Thymus extract has been shown to normalize the ratio of T-helper cells to suppressor cells, whether the ratio is low or high.[20,21] This effect is significant to CFS, as both increased and decreased helper/suppressor T-cell ratios have been noted in patients with CFS.

Thymus Extracts and Chronic Viral Infections   Thymus extracts may provide the answer to chronic infections, including CFS, by restoring healthy immune function. The ability of thymus extracts to treat and then reduce the number of recurrent infections was studied in groups of children with a history of recurrent respiratory tract infections. Double-blind studies revealed not only that orally administered thymus extracts were able to effectively eliminate infection, but that treatment over the course of a year significantly reduced the number of respiratory infections and significantly improved numerous immune parameters.[22] In addition, several studies have shown thymus extracts to be helpful in treating type B viral hepatitis, one of the hardest viruses for the body to throw off.[23,24]

Dosage of Thymus Extract   The proper dosage will vary from one manufacturer to another as there are no quality-control procedures or standards enforced in the glandular industry; it is left up to the individual company to adopt quality control and good manufacturing procedures.

From a practical view, products concentrated and standardized for polypeptide content are preferable to crude preparations. Based on current clinical research, the daily dose should be equivalent to 120 milligrams pure polypeptides with molecular weights less than 10,000, or roughly 500 milligrams of the crude polypeptide fraction. No side effects or adverse effects have been reported with the use of thymus preparations.

Plant-Based Medicines   Many herbs have shown remarkable effects in enhancing and modulating immune functions. It seems that modern research is upholding what herbal practitioners have known for thousands of years: herbs work with our body's systems to promote health. Chapter 11 details some of the more popular plant-based medicines to utilize in an attempt to enhance the immune system.

Chapter Summary

This chapter has described the immune system, its components, and natural ways to enhance its function. Perhaps the most important determinant of your immune status is your lifestyle. Maintaining a positive attitude, adopting a healthy lifestyle, reducing stress, following the dietary guidelines, and ensuring optimum levels of essential nutrients and antioxidants are critical to a healthy immune system. When additional support is necessary, preparations containing calf thymus tissue and various plant-based medicines can be extremely helpful in restoring healthy immune system function.

9

Chronic Fatigue and Adrenal Function

Have you ever been extremely tired and then all of a sudden felt a burst of energy? More than likely the sudden burst was due to the release of adrenaline from your adrenal glands, a pair of glands that lie on top of each kidney. If you have ever been suddenly frightened, you know how it feels to have adrenaline surge through your body. Adrenaline is there to give the body that extra energy boost to escape from danger.

In the less extreme case, adrenaline and other adrenal hormones regulate many body functions, including energy levels. When adrenal function is impaired, fatigue will result. There is now considerable evidence that many people with CFS have impaired adrenal function. Learning to deal with stress and supporting the adrenal glands are essential to the successful treatment of CFS in most cases. In order to have high energy levels, the adrenal glands must be working properly.

Stress and the Adrenals

Some basic control mechanisms in the body are geared toward counteracting the everyday stresses of life. However, if stress is extreme, unusual, or long-lasting, these control mechanisms can be quite harmful. Stress triggers a number of biological changes known collectively as the "general adaptation syndrome." The three phases of the general adaptation syndrome are alarm, resistance, and finally exhaustion.[1] These phases are controlled and regulated by the adrenal glands.

Alarm Reaction

The body's initial response to stress is the alarm reaction or "flight or fight" response. It is triggered by reactions in the brain which ultimately cause the adrenals to secrete adrenaline and other stress-related hormones. The fight or flight response is designed to counteract danger by mobilizing the body's resources for immediate physical activity. Your heart rate and force of contraction of the heart increases to provide blood to areas necessary for response to the stressful situation. Blood is shunted away from the skin and internal organs, except the heart and lungs, and the amount of blood supplying needed oxygen and glucose to the muscles and brain is increased. Your rate of breathing increases to supply necessary oxygen to the heart, brain, and exercising muscle. Sweat production increases to eliminate toxic compounds produced by the body and to lower body temperature. Production of digestive secretions is severely reduced, since digestive activity is not critical for counteracting stress. And blood sugar levels are increased dramatically as the liver dumps stored glucose into the bloodstream.

Resistance Reaction

While the fight or flight response is usually short-lived, the resistance reaction allows the body to continue fighting a stressor long after the effects of the fight or flight response have worn off. Corticosteroids secreted by the adrenal cortex are largely responsible for the resistance reaction. For example, the glucocorticoids stimulate the conversion of protein to energy so that the body has a large supply of energy long after glucose stores are depleted and the mineralocorticoids retain sodium to maintain an elevated blood pressure.

As well as providing the necessary energy and circulatory changes required to deal effectively with stress, the resistance reaction provides those changes required for meeting emotional crisis, performing strenuous tasks, and fighting infection. However, while the effects of adrenal cortex hormones are quite necessary when the body is faced with danger, prolongation of the resistance reaction or continued stress increases the risk of significant disease and results in the final stage of the general adaptation syndrome—exhaustion.

Exhaustion

Exhaustion may manifest by a total collapse of body function or a collapse of specific organs. Two major causes of exhaustion are loss of potassium ions and depletion of adrenal glucocorticoid hormones like cortisone.[1] When the cells of the body lose potassium they function less effectively and eventually die. When adrenal glucocorticoid stores become depleted hypoglycemia results, and cells of the body do not receive enough glucose or other nutrients.

Another cause of exhaustion is weakening of the organs. Prolonged stress places a tremendous load on many organ systems, especially the heart, blood vessels, adrenals, and immune system.

Healthy Adrenal Function

An abnormal adrenal response, either deficient or excessive hormone release, significantly alters an individual's response to stress. Healthy adrenal function is a key to dealing with stress. Often the adrenals become "exhausted" as a result of constant demands placed upon them. An individual with adrenal exhaustion will suffer from chronic fatigue and may complain of feeling "stressed out." They will typically have a reduced resistance to allergies and infection.

Atrophy or shrinking of the adrenal glands is a common side effect of continual stress and cortisone administration. Due to the importance of the adrenal glands, optimum health is dependent on optimum adrenal function.

Supporting the Adrenal Glands

One of the best ways to support the adrenal glands is by dealing with stress effectively by using techniques designed to reduce stress. Exercise and relaxation techniques such as meditation, prayer, biofeedback, and self-hypnosis are vital components of a stress-management program. While exercise is itself a physical stressor, it is a beneficial way to incorporate the fight or flight response as part of a daily routine. Regular exercise leads to an increased ability to cope with stress and reduces the risk of stress-related diseases.

Relaxation techniques seek to counteract the results of stress by inducing its opposite reaction—relaxation. Although an individual may relax by simply sleeping, watching television, or reading a book, relaxation techniques are designed specifically to produce the "relaxation response."[2] The physiological effects of the relaxation response are opposite to those seen with stress. The relaxation response is designed for repair, maintenance, and restoration of the body.

To achieve the relaxation response you can practice meditation, prayer, progressive relaxation, self-hypnosis, or biofeedback. The best relaxation technique for you is a totally individual choice. The important thing is that you set aside at least 5 to 10 minutes each day for relaxation. These sessions will also help remind you to breathe throughout the day in a relaxed effective manner.

Progressive relaxation is a popular technique based on a very simple procedure—comparing tension against relaxation. Maybe you are not aware of the sensation of relaxation. In progressive relaxation you will learn how it feels to relax by comparing relaxation to muscle tension.

You will first be asked to contract the muscle forcefully for 1 to 2 seconds then give way to a feeling of relaxation. Do this progressively through all the muscles of your body, and eventually a deep state of relaxation will result. Begin by contracting the muscles of the face and neck; hold the contraction for at least 1 to 2 seconds then relax the muscles. Next contract the upper arms and chest then relax, followed by the lower arms and hands. Repeat the process progressively down the body, contract then relax the abdomen, the buttocks, the thighs, the calves, and the feet. Repeat two or three times. This technique is often used in the treatment of anxiety and insomnia.

Progressive relaxation, deep breathing exercises, or some other stress reduction technique are important components of a healthy lifestyle. For your health and well-being, set aside at least 5 to 10 minutes each day just to relax.

Nourishing the Adrenal Glands

During periods of stress, to restore proper adrenal function, it is very useful to nourish the adrenal glands with the aid of various nutrients and herbal substances.

Foremost in the restoration or maintenance of proper adrenal function is to ensure adequate potassium levels within the body, by consuming foods rich in potassium and avoiding foods high in sodium. Most Americans have a potassium-to-sodium (K:Na) ratio of less than 1:2. This means most people ingest twice as much sodium as potassium.

Researchers recommend a dietary potassium-to-sodium ratio of greater than 5:1 to maintain health. This ratio is ten times higher than the average intake. However, even this may not be optimal. A natural diet rich in fruits and vegetables can produce a K:Na ratio greater than 50:1, as most fruits and vegetables have a K:Na ratio of at least 100:1. For example, here are the average K:Na ratios for several common fresh fruits and vegetables:

Carrots	75:1
Potatoes	110:1
Apples	90:1
Bananas	440:1
Oranges	260:1

To support the adrenals, daily intake of potassium should be at least 3 to 5 grams. Table 9.1 lists some foods having a high content of potassium.

Useful Nutrients

Vitamin C, vitamin B6, zinc, magnesium, and pantothenic acid are necessary nutrients for the manufacture of hormones by the adrenal glands. Supplementation of all of these nutrients at higher than RDA levels in the form of a high-potency multiple vitamin-mineral formula may be appropriate during periods of high stress or in individuals needing adrenal support.

Particularly important for optimum adrenal function is pantothenic acid. Pantothenic acid deficiency results in adrenal atrophy, which is characterized by fatigue, headache, sleep disturbance, nausea, and abdominal discomfort.[3] Pantothenic acid is found in whole grains, legumes, cauliflower, broccoli, salmon, liver, sweet potatoes, and tomatoes. It is a

Table 9.1 Potassium Content of Selected Foods

Milligrams (mg) per 100 grams edible portion (100 grams = 3.5 ounces)

Dulse	8,060	Cauliflower	295
Kelp	5,273	Watercress	282
Sunflower seeds	920	Asparagus	278
Wheat germ	827	Red cabbage	268
Almonds	773	Lettuce	264
Raisins	763	Cantaloupe	251
Parsley	727	Lentils, cooked	249
Brazil nuts	715	Tomato	244
Peanuts	674	Sweet potatoes	243
Dates	648	Papayas	234
Figs, dried	640	Eggplant	214
Avocados	604	Green peppers	213
Pecans	603	Beets	208
Yams	600	Peaches	202
Swiss chard	550	Summer squash	202
Soybeans, cooked	540	Oranges	200
Garlic	529	Raspberries	199
Spinach	470	Cherries	191
English walnuts	450	Strawberries	164
Millet	430	Grapefruit juice	162
Beans, cooked	416	Cucumbers	160
Mushrooms	414	Grapes	158
Potato with skin	407	Onions	157
Broccoli	382	Pineapple	146
Kale	378	Milk, whole	144
Bananas	370	Lemon juice	141
Meats	370	Pears	130
Winter squash	369	Eggs	129
Chicken	366	Apples	110
Carrots	341	Watermelon	100
Celery	341	Brown rice, cooked	70
Radishes	322		

SOURCE: "Nutritive Value of American Foods in Common Units," *U.S.D.A. Agriculture Handbook No. 456* good idea to take at least an additional 100 milligrams of pantothenic acid daily.

Adrenal Extracts

Oral adrenal extracts made from beef have been used in medicine since 1931.[4] Adrenal extracts may be made from the whole adrenal or just from the adrenal cortex. Whole adrenal extracts (usually in combination with essential nutrients for the adrenal glands) are most often used in cases of low adrenal function presenting as chronic fatigue, inability to cope with stress, and reduced resistance. Because extracts made from the adrenal cortex contain small amounts of corticosteroids, they are typically used as a "natural" cortisone in severe cases of allergy and inflammation (asthma, eczema, psoriasis, rheumatoid arthritis, etc.).

The dosage of adrenal extract will depend upon the quality and potency of the product. The best measure of an effective dose for either preparation may be the level of stimulation you experience. If a high-quality preparation is used, at higher dosages (for example, twice the label recommendation) you will notice a general stimulatory effect, including irritability, restlessness, and insomnia. I would suggest starting at one-third the recommended dosage on the label and slowly increasing your dosage every two days until you notice the stimulatory effect. Once you notice this, simply reduce your dosage to a level just below the level that will produce stimulation. As your adrenal glands rebuild, you will keep reducing the dosage until there comes a time when you do not require additional support.

Plant-Based Medicines

There are numerous herbs which support adrenal function. Most notable is ginseng. Both Siberian and Panax ginseng exert beneficial effects on adrenal function. Both of these herbs are discussed in Chapter 11.

Chapter Summary

The adrenal glands control many body functions and play a critical role in the resistance to stress and fatigue. If an individual has experienced a great deal of stress or has taken corticosteroids for a long period of time, the adrenal glands will shrink and not perform properly, causing them to experience chronic fatigue. In fact, low adrenal function is one of the hallmark features of CFS. We can support our adrenal glands by learning how to deal effectively with stress through the regular practice of relaxation techniques and exercise. In addition, the adrenal glands can be supported by eating a high-potassium diet along with taking nutritional supplements, adrenal extracts, and plant-based medicines such as ginseng.

10

Chronic Fatigue and Thyroid Function

As mentioned in Chapter 2, low thyroid function (hypo-thyroidism) is a common cause of chronic fatigue. Since the hormones of the thyroid gland regulate metabolism in every cell of the body, a deficiency of thyroid hormones can affect virtually all body functions. The degree of severity of symptoms in the adult range from extremely mild—deficiency states which are barely detectable (subclinical hypothyroidism)—to severe deficiency states which are life-threatening (myxedema).

How Common Is Hypothyroidism?

Most estimates on the rate of hypothyroidism in the general population are based on low levels of thyroid hormone levels in the blood. Using this method, a large number of people with mild hypothyroidism go undetected. Nonetheless, when blood levels of thyroid hormones are the criteria, it is esti-mated that 1% to 4% of the adult population have moderate to severe hypothyroidism, and another 10% to 12% have mild hypothyroidism.[1-3] The rate of hypothyroidism increases steadily with advancing age.

Manifestations of Adult Hypothyroidism

Since thyroid hormone affects every cell of the body, a deficiency will usually result in a large number of signs and symptoms. In addition to chronic fatigue, some of the common manifestations of hypothyroidism work on several body systems. Many of the symptoms that follow are common in CFS.

Metabolic   The metabolic manifestations of hypothyroidism are a general decrease in the rate of utilization of fat, protein, and carbohydrate. Moderate weight gain combined with cold intolerance is a common finding.

Cholesterol and triglyceride levels are increased in even the mildest forms of hypothyroidism. This elevation greatly increases the risk of serious cardiovascular disease. Studies have shown an increased rate of heart disease due to atherosclerosis in individuals with hypothyroidism.[4]

Hypothyroidism also leads to increased capillary permeability and slow lymphatic drainage. Often this will result in swelling of tissue (edema).

Endocrine   A variety of hormonal symptoms can exist in hypothyroidism. Perhaps the most common is a loss of libido (sexual drive) in men and menstrual abnormalities in women.

Women with mild hypothyroidism have prolonged and heavy menstrual bleeding, with a shorter menstrual cycle (time from the start of one period to the next). Infertility may also be a problem. If these women do become pregnant, miscarriages, premature deliveries, and stillbirths are common.

Rarely does a pregnancy terminate in normal labor and delivery in the hypothyroid woman.

Skin, Hair, and Nails   Dry, rough skin covered with fine superficial scales is seen in most hypothyroid individuals, and the hair is coarse, dry, and brittle. Hair loss can be quite severe. The nails become thin and brittle and typically show transverse grooves.

Psychological   The brain appears to be quite sensitive to low levels of thyroid hormone. Depression, along with weakness and fatigue, are usually the first symptoms of hypothyroidism.[5,6] Later, the hypothyroid individual will have difficulty concentrating and be extremely forgetful.

Muscular and Skeletal   Muscle weakness and joint stiffness are predominate features of hypothyroidism.[7] Some individuals with hypothyroidism may also experience muscle and joint pain, and tenderness.[9]

Cardiovascular   Hypothyroidism is thought to predispose one to atherosclerosis due to the increase in cholesterol and triglycerides.[8] Hypothyroidism can also cause hypertension, reduce the function of the heart, and reduce heart rate.

Other Manifestations   Shortness of breath, constipation, and impaired kidney function are other common symptoms of hypothyroidism.

Dietary Considerations in Hypothyroidism

Deficiency of any of a number of vitamins and minerals, especially iodine, but also including zinc, vitamins A, E, and C, and most B vitamins would result in lower levels of active thyroid hormone being produced.

Another dietary factor in hypothyroidism is that some foods contain substances which prevent the utilization of iodine. These foods are termed *goitrogens* and include such foods as turnips, cabbage, mustard, cassava root, soybeans, peanuts, pine nuts, and millet. Fortunately, cooking usually inactivates goitrogens.

Correcting Hypothyroidism

The medical treatment of hypothyroidism, in all but its mildest forms, involves the use of desiccated thyroid or synthetic thyroid hormone. Although synthetic hormones have become popular, many physicians (particularly naturopathic physicians) still prefer the use of desiccated natural thyroid, complete with all thyroid hormones. At this time, it appears that thyroid hormone replacement is necessary in the majority of people with hypothyroidism.

The thyroid extracts sold in health food stores are required by the Food and Drug Administration (FDA) to be thyroxine-free. However, it is nearly impossible to remove all the hormone from the gland. In other words, think of health-food-store thyroid preparations as milder forms of desiccated natural thyroid. If you have mild hypothyroidism, these preparations may provide enough support to help you with your thyroid problem. Follow the manufacturer's recommendations as provided on the product's label. Use your basal body temperature to determine effectiveness of the product. See Chapter 2 for a description of basal body temperature.

Exercise and Thyroid Function

Exercise is particularly important in a treatment program for hypothyroidism. Exercise stimulates thyroid gland secretion and increases tissue sensitivity to thyroid hormone. Many of the health benefits of exercise may be a result of improved thyroid function.

The health benefits of exercise are especially apparent in overweight hypothyroid individuals who are dieting (restricting food intake). A consistent effect of dieting is a decrease in the metabolic rate as the body strives to conserve fuel. Exercise has been shown to prevent the decline in metabolic rate in response to dieting.[9]

Chapter Summary

Hypothyroidism is common in the United States. Determining your basal body temperature is a functional test of thyroid function. In milder forms of hypothyroidism, commercial forms of thyroid available in health food stores may provide enough thyroid hormone and essential nutrients to support healthy thyroid function. In moderate to severe hypothyroidism, thyroid hormone replacement therapy is necessary.

11

Plant-Based Medicines
for Chronic Fatigue

M any different plant-based medicines are available to help relieve chronic fatigue and CFS. However, for many good reasons Siberian ginseng (*Eleutherococcus senticosus*) is emerging as the herb of choice. Siberian ginseng, Panax ginseng, St. John's wort (an herb useful in chronic fatigue because of its mood-elevating effects), and Shiitake mushroom extracts (useful in enhancing the immune system), are discussed in this chapter. In the Chapter Summary, you will find some practical guidelines to help you determine which plant-based medicine might be appropriate for you.

Siberian Ginseng

Modern interest in Siberian ginseng really began in Russia during the 1950s, as scientists began investigating substances which produce a "state of nonspecific resistance" on the body. Substances with this effect were termed *adaptogens*.

As defined by the famous Russian pharmacologist I. I. Brekhman in 1958, an adaptogen is a substance that: (1) must be innocuous and cause minimal disorders in the physiological functions of an organism; (2) must have a nonspecific action (it should increase the resistance to adverse influences by a wide range of physical, chemical, and biochemical factors); and (3) usually has a normalizing action irrespective of the direction of the pathologic state.[1,4]

Siberian Ginseng's Adaptogenic Activities

Siberian ginseng possesses a significant ability to increase nonspecific body resistance to stress, fatigue, and disease. It does this via a number of different mechanisms, but the key one may be inhibition of the fight or flight reaction (see Chapter 9). This antistress effect is thought to prevent much of the suppression of the immune system caused by stress.

Clinical Studies with Siberian Ginseng

Siberian ginseng root extract has been administered to more than 2,100 human subjects who were under stress, but otherwise healthy, in clinical trials for the purpose of evaluating its adaptogenic effects.[1] These studies indicated that Siberian ginseng: (1) increased the ability of humans to withstand many adverse physical conditions (heat, noise, motion, workload increase, exercise, and decompression); (2) increased mental alertness, work output, and energy levels; and (3) improved the quality of exertion under stressful conditions and athletic performance.

Siberian ginseng has also been administered to more than 2,200 human subjects in clinical trials for the purpose of evaluating its adaptogenic effect in disease states.[1] A variety of illnesses were included in these studies including angina, hypertension, hypotension, acute pyleonephritis, various types of neuroses, acute craniocerebral trauma, rheumatic heart disease, chronic bronchitis, and cancer.

Siberian Ginseng and Well-Being

Siberian ginseng appears to make people feel better. Not only stressed people feel better, Siberian ginseng has also consistently demonstrated an ability to increase the sense of general well-being in people experiencing a variety of psychological disturbances, including depression, insomnia, hypochondriasis, and various neuroses.

A possible explanation of this positive effect is improved balance among the various brain compounds like serotonin, dopamine, norepinephrine, and epinephrine. Siberian ginseng extract administered to rats has been shown to increase biogenic amine content in the brain, adrenals, and urine.[1] As individuals with CFS have been shown to have altered levels of these brain chemicals, it is likely that if Siberian ginseng does improve mood and energy levels in CFS it is via its ability to increase and improve the chemistry of the brain.

Siberian Ginseng and Immune Function

Siberian ginseng has been shown to exert a number of beneficial effects on immune function that may be useful in the treatment of CFS. In one double-blind study, 36 healthy subjects received either 10 milliliters of a Siberian ginseng fluid extract or a placebo daily for four weeks.[2] The group receiving the Siberian ginseng demonstrated significant improvements in a variety of immune system parameters. Most notable were a significant increase in T-helper cells and an increase in natural killer cell activity. Both of these effects could be put to good use in the treatment of CFS.

Dosage and Safety of Siberian Ginseng

Siberian ginseng is available in many different forms and strengths. Dosage depends upon which form you use. Here are the recommended dosages for the different commercially available forms. This dosage can be taken one to three times daily for periods up to 60 consecutive days, after which there is usually a two- to three-week interval between courses.

Dried root	2 to 4 grams
Tincture (1:5)	10 to 20 milliliters
Fluid extract (1:1)	2.0 to 4.0 milliliters
Solid (dry, powdered) extract (20:1 or standardized to contain greater than 1% eleutheroside E)	100 to 200 milligrams

Safety studies, as well as human clinical studies, demonstrate that Siberian ginseng extracts are very well tolerated and side effects are extremely uncommon. At higher dosages (a daily dose of six times the amounts listed above), however, side effects can include insomnia, irritability, melancholy, and anxiety. In individuals with rheumatic heart disease, pericardial pain, headaches, palpitations, and elevations in blood pressure have been reported.[1] Therefore, dosage should be monitored with caution in these individuals.

Panax Ginseng

Perhaps the most famous medicinal plant of China, Panax ginseng (Korean or Chinese ginseng) has been generally used as a tonic (alone or in combination with other herbs) for its revitalizing and energy-enhancing properties.

The active ingredients of Panax ginseng are compounds known as ginsenosides. The level and the ratio of ginsenosides determine the quality of ginseng. The type of ginsenosides are different in Panax ginseng and American ginseng (*Panax quinquefolius*). These differences are quite important yet subtle. Siberian ginseng contains no ginsenosides.

Research on Panax Ginseng

Since the 1950s, a great amount of research has been conducted worldwide to determine whether the healing properties attributed to Panax ginseng belong in the realm of legend or fact. Unfortunately, inconsistent results (due mostly to different procedures in the preparation of extracts, use of nonofficial parts of the plant, use of adulterants, and lack of quality control in the ginseng used) have made determination of Panax ginseng's true properties difficult. Nonetheless, enough good research exists to indicate that Panax ginseng produces results consistent with its near-legendary status, especially when high-quality extracts, standardized for active constituents, are used.[3,4]

Foremost among Panax ginseng's effects are its adaptogenic activities. According to tradition and scientific evidence, Panax ginseng possesses the necessary balancing, tonic, and antistress action to be termed an adaptogen. In fact, Panax ginseng is generally regarded as the most potent adaptogen.

The beneficial applications of Panax ginseng, like Siberian ginseng, are quite broad because of these adaptogenic qualities. Panax ginseng is especially effective in severely fatigued, debilitated, and feeble individuals. Like Siberian ginseng, human clinical studies with Panax ginseng have also shown it to increase feelings of energy; increase mental and physical performance; prevent the negative effects of stress and enhance the body's response to stress; offset some of the negative effects of cortisone; enhance liver function; and protect against radiation damage.[3,4]

One of the best studies demonstrating positive benefits involved the evaluation of the effect of Panax ginseng on nurses who had switched from day to night duty.[5] The nurses rated themselves for competence, mood, and general well-being, and were given a test for mental and physical performance along with blood cell counts and blood chemistry evaluations. The nurses who were administered Panax ginseng demonstrated better mental and physical performance and higher energy levels when compared with those receiving placebos. This study also highlights the fact that both men and women can benefit from Panax ginseng, contradicting the popular misconception that Panax ginseng is for "men only."

Panax Ginseng and Immune Function

Panax ginseng has been shown to enhance many immune functions including natural killer cell activity, interferon production, and macrophage activity. In one clinical study, three groups of 20 healthy volunteers were treated with capsules containing either 100 milligrams of aqueous extract of Panax ginseng (gp.A), 100 milligrams of lactose (gp.B), or 100 milligrams of a standardized extract (4% ginsenoside content) of Panax ginseng (gp.C).[6] All the volunteers took one capsule every 12 hours for eight weeks. Blood samples were withdrawn before beginning the treatment and again at weeks four and eight. A number of immune parameters were examined: the ability of neutrophils to move toward chemical toxins, the ability of neutrophils to engulf and destroy particulate matter (phagocytosis index, PHI, total lymphocytes (T3), T-helper (T4) subset, suppressor cells (T8) subset, and natural killer (NK) cells. Improvements noted by the subjects included improved neutrophil function, and increased PHI, total lymphocytes, T-helper cells, T4/T8 subsets, and NK cell activity. Although most of these effects were evident at four weeks, consistently greater effects were noted after eight weeks, implying that the beneficial effects of Panax ginseng on the immune system are cumulative.

Panax ginseng has an important effect on the so-called reticuloendothelial system. This part of the immune system is primarily composed of the macrophages of the liver (Kupffer cells), the spleen, and lymph nodes, and plays a major role in filtering the blood and removing particulate matter including viruses, bacteria, dead cells, cancer cells, and immune complexes. Another function of macrophages is to send strong messages to lymphocytes to seek out and destroy viruses, other microorganisms, and cancer cells. Panax ginseng administered to mice has resulted in a marked increase in the number and activities of macrophages.[3]

Choosing a Panax Ginseng Product

Many types and grades of ginseng and ginseng extracts are available, depending on the source, age, and parts of the root used, and the methods of preparation. Old, wild, well-formed roots are the most valued, while small roots of cultivated plants are considered the lowest grade. For largely economic purposes, the majority of ginseng in the American marketplace is derived from the lowest grade root, diluted with excipients, blended with adulterants, or totally devoid of ginsenosides.

High-quality ginseng extracts are available, however. The best preparations are those from the main root of plants between four and six years of age or extracts that have been standardized for ginsenoside content and ratio to ensure optimum pharmacological effect. The extracts are standardized not only for total ginsenoside content, but also for the ratio of ginsenoside $R_{b1}:R_{g1}$ (2:1 is considered ideal).

Dosage and Safety of Panax Ginseng

The use of standardized Panax ginseng preparations is recommended to ensure sufficient ginsenoside content, consistent benefits, and reduced risk of side effects. The typical dose (taken one to three times daily) for general tonic effects should contain a ginsenoside content of at least 15 milligrams. For example, for a standardized Panax ginseng extract containing a 7% saponin content calculated as ginsenoside R_{g1}, the standard dose would be 200 milligrams. As each individual's response to ginseng is unique, it is best to begin at lower doses and increase gradually. Again, the Russian approach for long-term administration is to use ginseng cyclically for a period of 15 to 20 days followed by a two-week interval without any ginseng. Care must be taken to observe possible ginseng toxicity.

Studies performed on standardized extracts of Panax ginseng have demonstrated the absence of side effects and toxicity.[3,4] Nonetheless, even when using standardized ginseng extracts, too much ginseng may cause a number of side effects including anxiety, irritability, nervousness, insomnia, hypertension, breast pain, and menstrual changes. If any of these side effects appear, the dosage should be reduced or the product discontinued.

St. John's Wort

St. John's wort (*Hypericum perforatum*) is a shrubby perennial plant native to many parts of the world including Europe and the United States. St. John's wort can be very useful in treating chronic fatigue—primarily by acting to improve the mood and relieve depression.

Recently, a tremendous amount of excitement was generated about St. John's wort after researchers demonstrated in a preliminary study that the St. John's wort components, hypericin and pseudohypericin, inhibit a variety of retroviruses including the retrovirus associated with AIDS (the human immuno-deficiency virus or HIV).[7] Although more research is needed to determine if St. John's wort is an appropriate recommendation in AIDS patients (based on its antiviral activity), it has been reported to improve the mood in AIDS patients. In one study, 65 out of 112 patients taking St. John's wort reported improved outlook, more energy, less fatigue, and feeling better.[8] Similar results have been noted in patients with CFS.

Researchers have discovered that components in St. John's wort alter brain chemistry in a way which improves the mood. These effects have been confirmed in clinical studies. A standardized extract of St. John's wort (0.125% hypericin) led to significant improvement in symptoms of anxiety, depression, and feelings of worthlessness.[9] In fact, its effectiveness in relieving depression has been shown to be greater than that produced by standard drugs used in depression, including amitriptyline (Elavil) and imiprimine (Trofinil). While these drugs are associated with significant side effects (most often drowsiness, dry mouth, constipation, and impaired urination), St. John's wort extract is not associated with any significant side effects. In addition to improving mood, the extract has been shown to greatly improve sleep quality; it was effective in relieving both insomnia and hypersomnia.

The dosage of St. John's wort extract used in most studies has been 300 milligrams (0.125% hypericin content) three times daily. Standardized extracts are preferable to other forms.

Shiitake Mushrooms

Many Americans consider mushrooms as simply non-nutritious garnish for salads or steaks, but in Asia mushrooms have been revered as potent medicines for thousands of years. During the past twenty years, mushrooms like the Shiitake mushroom (*Lentinus edodes*), have been extensively studied in Japan for their anticancer and immune-enhancing effects, largely as a result of anecdotal reports of their medicinal effects. This scientific investigation has led to the development of several mushroom extracts being approved as anticancer drugs by the Japanese government.

The immune-enhancing and anticancer effects of mushroom extracts are thought to be largely due to the polysaccharides. Polysaccharides are composed of individual sugar molecules chained together to form larger sugars and appear to activate macrophages and lymphocytes. Although some medicinal mushrooms like Shiitake and Reishi can be eaten freely in the diet, extracts are the preferred form for medicinal purposes. Because the cell walls of the mushrooms are made up of a high percentage of an indigestible fibrous material known as chitin, it is difficult for humans to gain all of the benefits from mushrooms unless they are cooked or processed in some manner.

Be aware of the difference between one product and another and realize that if you are simply taking a product composed of ground-up mushrooms, you are not likely to gain any benefit because the medicinal components of the mushrooms are locked inside an indigestible compartment. Cooking or processing in some manner is required in order to liberate the healing properties.

Medicinal Uses of Shiitake

The Shiitake mushroom is perhaps the most important medicinal mushroom, although the Reishi mushroom (*Ganoderma lucidum*) is a close second. The Shiitake mushroom is quite flavorful and nutritious, and is a mainstay in Japanese cuisine. However, eating huge amounts of the freshly-cooked mushrooms would be necessary to gain medicinal effects.

During the last 20 years, there has been a vast amount of research on Shiitake.[10] Most of the research has focused on its polysaccharide known as *lentinan*. Purified lentinan is an approved drug for cancer treatment in Japan. However, because lentinan is poorly absorbed when taken orally, lentinan must be injected to produce its effects. Lentinan has shown impressive results in prolonging the life span in cancer patients suffering from either breast, gastric, or colon cancers. Lentinan activates macrophages and other white blood cells, including natural killer cells.

Lentinan was shown to significantly increase natural killer cells by more than 300% in patients with CFS and greatly improved feelings of well-being including increased energy levels.[11] However, it must be pointed out that the lentinan was administered by injection at a dose of 1 milligram a day, every other day.

Because lentinan does not seem to be very effective when given orally, researchers have investigated other Shiitake polysaccharides and extracts for oral use. One of the most promising Shiitake extracts is known as KS-2. KS-2 is produced from the alcohol extract of the mycelium. What separates KS-2 from other mushroom polysaccharides is its chemical structure. KS-2 is called a *peptidomannan*. It is composed of a polysaccharide component bound to amino acids. Evidently, the binding of the polysaccharide to the amino acids facilitates oral absorption.[12,13]

KS-2 activates macrophages and induces the body to produce interferon—two very important actions in the treatment of CFS.

The KS-2 extract from Shiitake may prove to be the best for oral use because of its high oral bioavailability, combined with its powerful immune-enhancing effects. The dosage for KS-2 is 75 to 150 milligrams three times daily. Because the effects of lentinan have been shown to wear off after eight weeks of use, it is best to use KS-2 for short periods of time. Save its use for acute flare-ups of chronic viral infections, including chronic Epstein–Barr and Herpes, as well as in acute infectious conditions.

Chapter Summary

Plant-based medicines are useful allies in the battle against fatigue. There are many herbs to choose from. Those presented in this chapter—Siberian ginseng, Panax ginseng,

St. John's wort, and medicinal mushrooms—are perhaps the most beneficial, besides being the most popular. Here are some practical guidelines to help you determine which herbs may work best for you.

If needed, these plant-based medicines can be used simultaneously. The down side to this is cost. In addition, use of all of these plant-based medicines is usually not indicated.

I will use KS-2 in the initial treatment of CFS. Treatment with KS-2 is short-term, about four to eight weeks, because the body appears to build up a tolerance to the immune stimulation. At least two weeks between treatment courses appears to be necessary, to allow the body time to respond once again to the treatment.

I will use St. John's wort if the chronic fatigue appears to be caused primarily by underlying depression or if a person has poor sleep quality. Although St. John's wort may have some antiviral activity, I only use it for its mood-elevating effects and its ability to improve sleep quality.

Now, what about the ginsengs? Which one do I use? Most often Siberian ginseng, because in the treatment of chronic fatigue I tend to recommend a product which contains Siberian ginseng and a liquid liver extract (see Chapter 7). I rarely find that additional Siberian ginseng is required, but occasionally I may prescribe a supplemental dosage.

I tend to reserve the use of Panax ginseng for individuals who are severely debilitated, most often due to a long-standing illness or long-term use of corticosteroids.

Putting It All Together

12

The Energy Prescription

R emember, your energy level as well as your emotional
state is determined by two primary factors—internal
focus and physiology. The techniques I recommend for max-
imizing energy levels focus on improving either your mind
and attitude or your physiology. The goal of this final chapter
is to help you prioritize your symptoms, and then implement
the applicable measures detailed in previous chapters. Here
are seven steps to take toward higher energy and an end to
fatigue.

Step 1. Mind and Attitude

The first step on the way to having an abundance of
energy is *believing that you can* have an abundance of
energy. Follow the guidelines and techniques given in
Chapter 3 and the stress-management techniques in
Chapter 9.

Step 2. Diet

Track down and control food allergies and follow the
dietary guidelines given in Chapter 4.

Step 3. Breathing, Posture, and Bodywork

Breathe deeply and hold your body in a posture that is reflective of high energy. Find a good bodywork therapist and begin getting regular bodywork.

Step 4. Exercise

Start a regular exercise program. Go slow and easy at first, but eventually your increased energy levels will allow you to do more and more.

Step 5. Nutritional Supplements

Take a good multiple vitamin-mineral formula, and extra amounts of vitamin C and magnesium. Consider taking a liquid (hydrolyzed) liver extract.

Step 6. Specific Body Functions

You may need to support or enhance certain body functions.

- If you need additional liver support, take a lipotropic formula and follow the other recommendations given in Chapter 7.

- If you need additional immune support, take a high-quality thymus extract, extra vitamin C, and beta-carotene, and use Siberian ginseng (long-term) and KS-2 (short-term) to bolster the immune system.

- If you need adrenal support, make sure you are dealing with stress effectively and getting enough potassium in your diet. Consider trying either an adrenal extract or Siberian ginseng to support adrenal function.

- If you have hypothyroidism, follow the recommendations given in Chapter 10.

- If depression is a problem, take St. John's wort extract.

- If you have poor sleep quality, insomnia, or hypersomnia, take St. John's wort extract.

Step 7. Siberian or Panax Ginseng
The ginsengs are fantastic energy-enhancing herbs that exert many beneficial effects. Follow the guidelines given in Chapter 11.

If you follow these seven steps, you will avoid taking a lot of unnecessary medicines and pills. The program outlined in this book is designed to be as cost-effective as possible, while still providing the benefits you need. Fortunately, some of the best methods for increasing your energy levels are free— positive mind and attitude, deep breathing, and good posture. And, if you follow the dietary guidelines you will be providing tremendous nutritional support for many key body functions, including the liver and immune system.

I am confident that my comprehensive program will significantly improve your energy levels and your health. But if you follow these recommendations and still do not experience freedom from fatigue, I strongly urge you to consult a naturopathic physician (N.D.) or holistic medical doctor (M.D. or D.O.). There are a number of special techniques not discussed in this book that doctors in these fields can utilize to help you gain more energy. To find a physician in your area call or write:

The American Association of Naturopathic Physicians
P.O. Box 20386
Seattle, WA 98102
(206) 323–7610

or

The American Holistic Medical Association
4101 Lake Boone Trail #201
Raleigh, NC 26707
(919) 787–5146

References

Chapter 1: What Is Chronic Fatigue Syndrome?

1. Holmes GP, et al.: Chronic fatigue syndrome: A working case definition. Ann Int Med 108:387–9, 1988.

2. Bates DW, et al.: Prevalence of fatigue and chronic fatigue syndrome in a primary care practice. Arch Int Med 2759–65, 1993.

3. Shafran SD: The chronic fatigue syndrome. Am J Med 90:731–9, 1991.

4. Kyle DV and Deshazo RD: Chronic fatigue syndrome: A conundrum. Am J Med Sci 303:28–34, 1992.

5. Komaroff AL: Chronic fatigue syndromes: Relationship to chronic viral infections. J Virol Meth 21:3–10, 1988.

6. Jones JF, et al.: Evidence for active Epstein–Barr virus infection in patients with persistent unexplained illness: Elevated anti-early antigen antibodies. Ann Int Med 102:1–7, 1985.

7. Straus SE, et al.: Persisting illness and fatigue in adults with evidence of Epstein–Barr virus infection. Ann Int Med 102:7–16, 1985.

8. Holmes GP, Kaplan JE, Stewart JA, et al.: A cluster of patients with a chronic mononucleosis-like syndrome. Is Epstein–Barr virus the cause? JAMA 257:2297–302, 1987.

9. Caligiuri M, et al.: Phenotypic and functional deficiency of natural killer cells in patients with chronic fatigue syndrome. J Immunol 139:3306–13, 1987.

10. Gupta S and Vayuvegula B: A comprehensive immunological analysis in chronic fatigue syndrome. Scand J Immunol 33:319–27, 1991.

11. Komaroff Al and Goldenberg D: The chronic fatigue syndrome: Definition, current studies and lessons for fibromyalgia research. J Rheumatol 16(Suppl. 19):23–7, 1989.

Chapter 2: Diagnosing the Causes of Chronic Fatigue Syndrome

1. Holmes TH and Rahe RH: The social readjustment scale. J Psychosomatic Res 11:213–8, 1967.

2. Seaton A, Jeelinek EH, and Kennedy P: Major neurological disease and occupational exposure to organic solvents. Quart J Med 305:707–12, 1992.

3. Rutter M and Russell-Jones R (eds): Lead versus Health: Sources and Effects of Low-Level Lead Exposure. John Wiley, New York, 1983.

4. Rowe AH and Rowe A, Jr.: Food Allergy: Its Manifestations and Control and the Elimination Diets: A Compendium. Charles C. Thomas, Springfield, IL, 1972.

5. Breneman JC: Basics of Food Allergy. Charles C. Thomas, Springfield, IL, 1977.

6. Barnes BO and Galton L: Hypothyroidism: The Unsuspected Illness. Thomas Crowell, New York, 1976.

7. Langer SE and Scheer JF: Solved: The Riddle of Illness. Keats, New Canaan, CT, 1984.

8. Gold M, Pottash A, and Extein I: Hypothyroidism and depression, evidence from complete thyroid function evaluation. JAMA 245:1919–22, 1981.

9. Chalew SA, et al.: Diagnosis of reactive hypoglycemia: pitfalls in the use of the oral glucose tolerance test. Southern Medical J 79:285–7, 1986.

10. Chalew SA, et al.: The use of the plasma epinephrine response in the diagnosis of idiopathic postprandial syndrome. JAMA 251: 612–5, 1984.

11. Hadji-Georgopoulus A, et al.: Elevated hypoglycemic index and late hyperinsulinism in symptomatic postprandial hypoglycemia. J Clin Endocrinol Metab 50:371–6, 1980.

12. Fabrykant M: The problem of functional hyperinsulinism on functional hypoglycemia attributed to nervous causes. 1. Laboratory and clinical correlations. Metab 4:469–79, 1955.

13. Anderson RA, Polansky MM, Bryden NA, et al.: Effects of supplemental chromium on patients with symptoms of reactive hypoglycemia. Metab 36:351–5, 1987.

Chapter 3: Tuning Up the Mind and Attitude

1. White LB, Tursky B, and Schwartz G (eds): Placebos: Theory, Research and Mechanisms. Guilford, New York, 1985.

2. Vollhardt LT: Psychoneuroimmunology: A literature review. Am J Orthopsychiatry 61:35–47, 1991.

3. Kiecolt-Glaser JK and Glaser R: Psychoneuroimmunology: Can psychological interventions modulate immunity? J Consult Clin Psychol 60:569–75, 1992.

4. Bartrop RW, et al.: Depressed lymphocyte function after bereavement. Lancet i:834–6, 1977.

5. Schleifer SJ, et al.: Suppression of lymphocyte stimulation following bereavement. JAMA 250:374–7, 1983.

6. Cousins N: Anatomy of an Illness. Bantam, New York, 1979.

7. Dillon KM and Minchoff B: Positive emotional states and enhancement of the immune system. Int J Psychiatry Med 15:13–7, 1986.

8. Martin RA and Dobbin JP: Sense of humor, hassles, and immunoglobulin A: Evidence for a stress-moderating effect of humor. Int J Psychiatry Med 18:93–105, 1988.

9. Irwin M, et al.: Reduction of immune function in life stress and depression. Biol Psych 27:22–30, 1990.

10. O'Leary A: Stress, emotion, and human immune function. Psychol Bull 108:363–82, 1990.

11. Peterson C: Explanatory style as a risk factor for illness. Cog Ther Res 12:117–30, 1988.

12. Peterson C, Seligman M, and Valliant G: Pessimistic explanatory style as a risk factor for physical illness: A thirty-five year longitudinal study. J Person Soc Psych 55:23–7, 1988.

13. Seligman ME: Learned Optimism. Alfred A. Knopf, New York, 1990.

Chapter 4: Dietary Guidelines

1. Chou T. Wake up and smell the coffee. Caffeine, coffee, and the medical consequences. West J Med 157:544–53, 1992.

2. Hughes JR, et al.: Caffeine self-administration, withdrawal, and adverse effects among coffee drinkers. Arch Gen Psych 48:611–7, 1991.

3. Estler CJ, Ammon HP, and Herzog C: Swimming capacity of mice after prolonged treatment with psychostimulants. I. Effects of caffeine on swimming performance and cold stress. Psychopharmacol 58:161–6, 1978.

4. Greden JF, et al.: Anxiety and depression associated with caffeinism among psychiatric inpatients. Am J Psychiatry 135:963–6, 1978.

5. Stich HF: Teas and tea components as inhibitors of carcinogen formation in model systems and man. Prev Med 21:377–84, 1992.

6. Editorial: Statement on hypoglycemia. JAMA 223:682, 1972.

7. Cahill GF and Soelder JS: A non-editorial on non-hypoglycemia. N Engl J Med 291:905–6, 1974.

8. Hofeldt FD: Patients with bona fide meal-related hypoglycemia should be treated primarily with dietary restriction of refined carbohydrate. Endocrinol Metab Clin North Am 18:185–201, 1989.

9. Sanders LR, et al.: Refined carbohydrate as a contributing factor in reactive hypoglycemia. Southern Medical J 75:1072–5, 1982.

10. Reaven GM: Role of insulin resistance in human disease. Diabetes 37:1595–1607, 1988.

11. National Research Council: Diet and Health. Implications for Reducing Chronic Disease Risk. National Academy Press, Washington, DC, 1989.

12. Winokur A, et al.: Insulin resistance after glucose-tolerance testing in patients with major depression. Am J Psychiatry 145:325–30, 1988.

13. Wright JH, et al.: Glucose metabolism in unipolar depression. Br J Psychiatry 132:386–93, 1978.

14. Schauss AG: Nutrition and behavior: Complex interdisciplinary research. Nutr Health 3:9–37, 1984.

15. Jenkins DJA, et al.: Glycemic index of foods: A physiological basis for carbohydrate exchange. Am J Clin Nutr 24:362–6, 1981.

16. Truswell AS: Glycemic index of foods. Eur J Clin Nutr 46 (Supplement 2):S91–101, 1992.

17. Koivisto VA and Yki-Jarvinen H: Fructose and insulin sensitivity in patients with type 2 diabetes. J Int Med 233:145–53, 1993.

18. Gregersen S, et al.: Glycaemic and insulinaemic responses to orange and apple compared with white bread in non-insulin dependent diabetic subjects. Eur J Clin Nutr 46:301–3, 1992.

19. Block G: Dietary guidelines and the results of food consumption surveys. Am J Clin Nutr 53:356S–7S, 1991.

20. Wald NJ, et al.: Serum beta-carotene and subsequent risk of cancer: Results from the BUPA study. Br J Cancer 57:428–33, 1988.

21. Harris RWC, et al.: A case-control study of dietary carotene in men with lung cancer and in men with other epithelial cancers. Nutr Cancer 15:63–8, 1991.

22. Peto R, et al.: Can dietary beta-carotene materially reduce human cancer rates? Nature 290:201–8, 1981.

23. Rogers AE and Longnecker MP: Biology of disease: Dietary and nutritional influences on cancer: A review of epidemiologic and experimental data. Lab Invest 59:729–59, 1988.

24. Konowalchuk J and Speirs JI: Antiviral effect of apple beverages. Appl Envir Microbiol 36:798–801, 1978.

25. Shils ME and Young VR: Modern Nutrition in Health and Disease, 7th edition. Lea and Febiger, Philadelphia, 1988.

26. White PL and Selvey N: Nutritional Qualities of Fresh Fruits and Vegetables. Futura Publishing, Mount Kisco, NY, 1974.

27. Stanto JL and Keast DR: Serum cholesterol, fat intake, and breakfast consumption in the United States adult population. J Am Coll Nutr 8:567–72, 1989.

28. Furia T (ed): CRC Handbook of Food Additives, vols 1 and 2. CRC Press, Boca Raton, FL, 1980.

Chapter 5: Physical Care of the Body

1. Pollack ML, Wilmore JH, and Fox SM: Exercise in Health and Disease. WB Saunders, Philadelphia, 1984.

2. Farmer ME, Locke BZ, Mosciki EK, et al.: Physical activity and depressive symptomatology: The NHANES 1 epidemiologic follow-up study. Am J Epidemiol 1328:1340–51, 1988.

3. Fiatarone MA, et al.: The effect of exercise on natural killer cells activity in young and old subjects. J Gerontol 44:M37–45, 1989.

4. Makinnon LT: Exercise and natural killer cells: What is their relationship? Sports Med 7:141–9, 1989.

5. Xusheng S, Yugi X, and Yunjian X: Determination of E-rosette-forming lymphocytes in aged subjects with tai chi quan exercise. Int J Sport Med 10:217–9, 1989.

6. Fitzgerald L: Exercise and the immune system. Immunol Today 9:337–9, 1988.

Chapter 6: Nutritional Supplementation

1. Block G, et al.: Vitamin supplement use, by demographic characteristics. Am J Epidemiol 127:297–309, 1988.

2. National Research Council: Diet and Health. Implications for Reducing Chronic Disease Risk. National Academy Press, Washington, DC, 1989.

3. National Research Council: Recommended Dietary Allowances, 10th edition. National Academy Press, Washington, DC, 1989.

4. Chandra RK: Effect of vitamin and trace-element supplementation on immune responses and infection in elderly subjects. Lancet 340:1124–7, 1992.

5. Shils ME and Young VR: Modern Nutrition in Health and Disease, 7th edition. Lea and Febiger, Philadelphia, 1988.

6. Cheraskin E: Vitamin C—Who Needs It? Arlington Press, Birmingham, AL, 1993.

7. Hemila H: Vitamin C and the common cold. Br J Nutr 67:3–16, 1992.

8. Scott J: On the biochemical similarities of ascorbic acid and interferon. J Theor Biol 98:235–8, 1982.

9. Ginter E: Optimum intake of vitamin C for the human organism. Nutr Health 1:66–77, 1982.

10. Pauling L: Vitamin C and the Common Cold. Freeman, San Francisco, 1970.

11. Cathcart RF: The third face of vitamin C. J Orthomol Med 7:197–200, 1992.

12. Morgan KJ, Stampley GL, and Zabik ME: Magnesium and calcium dietary intakes of the U.S. population. J Am Coll Nutr 4:195–206, 1985.

13. Cox IM, Campbell MJ, and Dowson D: Red blood cell magnesium and chronic fatigue syndrome. Lancet 337:757–60, 1991.

14. Ahlborg H, Ekelund LG, and Nilsson CG: Effect of potassium-magnesium aspartate on the capacity for prolonged exercise in man. Acta Physiol Scand 74:238–45, 1968.

15. Hicks JT: Treatment of fatigue in general practice: A double-blind study. Clin Med Jan:85–90, 1964.

16. Friedlander HS: Fatigue as a presenting symptom: Management in general practice. Current Ther Res 4:441–9, 1962.

17. Shaw DL: Management of fatigue: A physiologic approach. Am J Med Sci 243:758–69, 1962.

18. Gullestad L, et al.: Oral versus intravenous magnesium supplementation in patients with magnesium deficiency. Magnes Trace Elem 10:11–6, 1991.

19. Lindberg JS, et al.: Magnesium bioavailability from magnesium citrate and magnesium oxid. J Am Coll Nutr 9:48–55, 1990.

20. Cook JD and Lynch SR: The liabilities of iron deficiency. Blood 68:803–9, 1986.

21. Viteri FE and Torun B: Anaemia and physical work capacity. Clin Haematol 3:609–26, 1974.

22. Gardner GW, et al.: Physical work capacity and metabolic stress in subjects with iron deficiency anemia. Am J Clin Nutr 30:910–7, 1977.

23. Krause MV and Mahan KL: Food, Nutrition and Diet Therapy, 7th edition. WB Saunders, Philadelphia, 1984.

24. Jacobs AM and Owen GM: The effect of age on iron absorption. J Gerontol 24:95–6, 1969.

25. Bezwoda W, et al.: The importance of gastric hydrochloric acid in the absorption of nonheme iron. J Lab Clin Med 92:108–16, 1978.

26. Nagai K: A study of the excretory mechanism of the liver—Effect of liver hydrolysate on BSP excretion. Jap J Gastroenterol 67:633–8, 1970.

27. Ohbayashi A, Akioka T, and Tasaki H: A study of effects of liver hydrolysate on hepatic circulation. J Ther 54:1582–5, 1972.

28. Sanbe K, et al.: Treatment of liver disease—With particular reference to liver hydrolysates. Jap J Clin Exp Med 50:2665–76, 1973.

29. Fujisawa K, et al.: Therapeutic effects of liver hydrolysate preparation on chronic hepatitis—A double-blind, controlled study. Asian Med J 26:497–526, 1984.

Chapter 7: Chronic Fatigue and Liver Function

1. Regenstein L: America the Poisoned. Acropolis, Washington, DC, 1982.

2. Rutter M and Russell-Jones R (eds): Lead versus Health: Sources and Effects of Low-Level Lead Exposure. John Wiley, New York, 1983.

3. Klein A, et al.: The effect of nonviral liver damage on the T-lymphocyte helper/suppressor ratio. Clin Immunol Immunopathol 46:214–20, 1988.

4. Abe F, Nagata S, and Hotchi M: Experimental candidiasis in liver injury. Mycopathol 100:37–42, 1987.

5. Flora SJS, Singh S, and Tandon SK: Prevention of lead intoxication by vitamin B complex. Z Ges Hyg 30:409–11, 1984.

6. Shakman RA: Nutritional influences on the toxicity of environmental pollutants: A review. Arch Env Health 28:105–33, 1974.

7. Flora SJS, et al.: Protective role of trace metals in lead intoxication. Toxicol Lett 13:51–6, 1982.

8. Padova C, et al.: S-adenosyl-L-methionine antagonizes oral contraceptive-induced bile cholesterol supersaturation in healthy women: Preliminary report of a controlled randomized trial. Am J Gastroenterol 79:941–4, 1984.

9. Frezza M, et al.: Reversal of intrahepatic cholestasis of pregnancy in women after high dose S-adenosyl-L-methionine (SAMe) administration. Hepatol 4:274–8, 1984.

10. Bombardieri G, et al.: Effects of S-adenosyl-methionine (SAMe) in the treatment of Gilbert's syndrome. Current Ther Res 37:580–5, 1985.

11. Wisniewska-Knypl J, et al.: Protective effect of methionine against vinyl chloride-mediated depression of non-protein sulfhydryls and cytochrome P-450. Toxicol Lett 8:147–52, 1981.

12. Barak AJ, et al.: Dietary betaine promotes generation of hepatic S-adenosylmethionine and protects the liver from ethanol-induced fatty infiltration. Alcohol Clin Exp Res 17:552–5, 1993.

13. Zeisel SH, et al.: Choline, an essential nutrient for humans. FASEB J 5:2093–8, 1991.

14. Ballatori N and Clarkson TW: Dependence of biliary excretion of inorganic mercury on the biliary transport of glutathione. Biochemical Pharmacol 33:1093–8, 1984.

15. Murakami M and Webb MA: A morphological and biochemical study of the effects of L-cysteine on the renal uptake and nephrotoxicity of cadmium, Br J Exp Pathol 62:115–30, 1981.

16. Baker DH and Czarnecki-Maulden GL: Pharmacologic role of cysteine in ameliorating or exacerbating mineral toxicities. J Nutr 117:1003–10, 1987.

17. Ruffmann R and Wendel A: GSH rescue by N-acetylcysteine. Klin Wochenschr 69:857–62, 1991.

18. Hikino H, et al.: Antihepatotoxic actions of flavonolignans from *Silybum marianum* fruits. Planta Medica 50:248–50, 1984.

19. Vogel G, et al.: Studies on pharmacodynamics, site and mechanism of action of silymarin, the antihepatotoxic principle from *Silybum marianum* (L.) Gaert. Arzneim Forsch 25:179–85, 1975.

20. Wagner H: Antihepatotoxic flavonoids. In: Plant Flavonoids in Biology and Medicine: Biochemical, Pharmacological, and Structure-Activity Relationships. Cody V, Middleton E, and Harbourne JB (eds). Alan R. Liss, New York, 1986, pp. 545–58.

21. Valenzuela A, et al.: Selectivity of silymarin on the increase of the glutathione content in different tissues of the rat. Planta Medica 55:420–2, 1989.

22. Sarre H: Experience in the treatment of chronic hepatopathies with silymarin. Arzneim Forsch 21:1209–12, 1971.

23. Canini F, Bartolucci, Cristallini E, et al.: Use of silymarin in the treatment of alcoholic hepatic steatosis. Clin Ter 114:307–14, 1985.

24. Salmi HA and Sarna S: Effect of silymarin on chemical, functional, and morphological alteration of the liver. A double-blind controlled study. Scand J Gastroent 17:417–21, 1982.

25. Boari C, et al.: Occupational toxic liver diseases. Therapeutic effects of silymarin. Min Med 72:2679–88, 1985.

26. Ferenci P, et al.: Randomized controlled trial of silymarin treatment in patients with cirrhosis of the liver. J Hepatol 9:105–13, 1989.

27. Imamura M and Tung T: A trial of fasting cure for PCB-poisoned patients in Taiwan. Am J Ind Med 5:147–53, 1984.

Chapter 8: Chronic Fatigue and Immune Function

1. Fridkin M and Najjar VA: Tuftsin: Its chemistry, biology, and clinical potential. Crit Rev Biochem Mol Biol 24:1–40, 1989.

2. Rastogi A, et al.: Augmentation of human natural killer cells by splenopentin analogs. FEBS Lett 317:93–5, 1993.

3. Minter MM: Agranulocytic angina: Treatment of a case with fetal calf spleen. Texas State J Med 2:338–43, 1933.

4. Gray GA: The treatment of agranulocytic angina with fetal calf spleen. Texas State J Med 29:366–9, 1933.

5. Moldofsky H, et al.: The relationship of interleukin-1 and immune functions to sleep in humans. Psychosomatic Med 48:309–18, 1986.

6. Kusaka Y, Kondou H, and Morimoto K: Healthy lifestyles are associated with higher natural killer cell activity. Prev Med 21:602–15, 1992.

7. Nekachi K and Imai K: Environmental and physiological influences on human natural killer cell activity in relation to good health practices. Jap J Cancer Res 83:789–805, 1992.

8. National Research Council: Diet and Health. Implications for Reducing Chronic Disease Risk. National Academy Press, Washington, DC, 1989.

9. Palmblad J, Hallberg D, and Rossner S: Obesity, plasma lipids and polymorphonuclear (PMN) granulocyte functions. Scand J Heamatol 19:293–303, 1977.

10. Sanchez A, et al.: Role of sugars in human neutrophilic phagocytosis. Am J Clin Nutr 26:1180–4, 1973.

11. Ringsdorf W, Cheraskin E, and Ramsay R: Sucrose, neutrophil phagocytosis and resistance to disease. Dent Surv 52:46–8, 1976.

12. Bernstein J, et al.: Depression of lymphocyte transformation following oral glucose ingestion. Am J Clin Nutr 30:613, 1977.

13. Mann G and Newton P: The membrane transport of ascorbic acid. Ann NY Acad Sci 258:243–51, 1975.

14. Brown MB (ed): Present Knowledge in Nutrition, 6th edition. Nutrition Foundation, Washington, DC, 1990.

15. Beisel WR: Single nutrients and immunity. Am J Clin Nutr 35:S417–68, 1982.

16. Alexander M, Newmark H, and Miller R: Oral beta-carotene can increase the number of OKT4+ cells in human blood. Immunol Lett 9:221–4, 1985.

17. Vojdani A and Ghoneum M: In vivo effect of ascorbic acid on enhancement of human natural killer cell activity. Nutr Res 13:753–64, 1993.

18. Dardenne M, et al.: Contribution of zinc and other metals to the biological activity of the serum thymic factor. Proc Natl Acad Sci 79:5370–3, 1982.

19. Bogden JD, et al.: Zinc and immunocompetence in the elderly: Baseline data on zinc nutriture and immunity in unsupplemented subjects. Am J Clin Nutr 46:101–9, 1987.

20. Cazzola P, Mazzanti P, and Bossi G: In vivo modulating effect of a calf thymus acid lysate on human T lymphocyte subsets and CD4+/CD8+ ratio in the course of different diseases. Current Ther Res 42:1011–7, 1987.

21. Kouttab NM, Prada M, and Cazzola P: Thymomodulin: Biological properties and clinical applications. Med Oncol Tumor Pharmacother 6:5–9, 1989.

22. Fiocchi A, et al.: A double-blind clinical trial for the evaluation of the therapeutic effectiveness of a calf thymus derivative (Thymomodulin) in children with recurrent respiratory infections. Thymus 8:831–9, 1986.

23. Galli M, et al.: Attempt to treat acute type B hepatitis with an orally administered thymic extract (Thymomodulin): Preliminary results. Drugs Exp Clin Res 11:665–9, 1985.

24. Bortolotti F, et al.: Effect of an orally administered thymic derivative, Thymodulin, in chronic type B hepatitis in children. Current Ther Res 43:67–72, 1988.

Chapter 9: Chronic Fatigue and Adrenal Function

1. Seyle H: Stress in Health and Disease. Buttersworth, London, 1976.

2. Benson H: The Relaxation Response. William Morrow, New York, 1975.

3. Nutrition Foundation: Present Knowledge in Nutrition, 5th edition. Nutrition Foundation, Washington, DC, 1984.

4. Britton SW and Silvette H: Further experiments on cortico-adrenal extract: Its efficacy by mouth. Science 74:440–1, 1931.

Chapter 10: Chronic Fatigue and Thyroid Function

1. Mazzaferri EL: Adult hypothyroidism. Postgrad Med 79:64–72, 1986.

2. Drinka PJ and Nolten WE: Review: Subclinical hypothyroidism in the elderly: To treat or not to treat? Am J Med Sci 295:125–8, 1988.

3. Banovac K, Zakarija M, and McKenzie JM: Experience with routine thyroid function testing: Abnormal results in "normal" populations. J Flor Med Assoc 72:835–9, 1985.

4. Althaus U, Staub JJ, Ryff-De Leche A, et al.: LDL/HDL-changes in subclinical hypothyroidism: Possible risk factors for coronary heart disease. Clin Endocrinol 28:157–63, 1988.

5. Gold M, Pottash A, and Extein I: Hypothyroidism and depression, evidence from complete thyroid function evaluation. JAMA 245:1919–22, 1981.

6. Joffe R, Roy-Byrne P, and Udhe T: Thyroid function and affective illness: A reappraisal. Biol Psychiatry 19:1685–91, 1984.

7. Krupsky M, et al.: Musculoskeletal symptoms as a presenting sign of long-standing hypothyroidism. Isr J Med Sci 23:1110–3, 1987.

8. Turnbridge WMG, Evered DC, and Hall R: Lipid profiles and cardiovascular disease in the Wickham area with particular reference to thyroid failure. Clin Endocrinol 7:495–508, 1977.

9. Lennon D, et al.: Diet and exercise training effects on resting metabolic rate. Int J Obesity 9:39–47, 1985.

Chapter 11: Plant-Based Medicines for Chronic Fatigue

1. Farnsworth NR, et al.: Siberian ginseng (*Eleutherococcus senticosus*): Current status as an adaptogen. Econ Med Plant Res 1:156–215, 1985.

2. Bohn B, Nebe CT, and Birr C: Flow-cytometric studies with *Eleutherococcus senticosus* extract as an immunomodulatory agent. Arzneim Forsch 37:1193–6, 1987.

3. Hikino H: Chapter 11: Traditional remedies and modern assessment: The case of ginseng. In: The Medicinal Plant Industry. Wijeskera ROB (ed). CRC Press, Boca Raton, FL, 1991, pp. 149–66.

4. Shibata S, et al.: Chemistry and pharmacology of Panax. Econ Med Plant Res 1:217–84, 1985.

5. Hallstrom C, Fulder S, and Carruthers M: Effect of ginseng on the performance of nurses on night duty. Comp Med East West 6:277–82, 1982.

6. Scaglione F et al.: Immunomodulatory effects of two extracts of Panax ginseng C.A. Meyer. Drugs Exp Clin Res 16:537–42, 1990.

7. Meruelo D, et al.: Therapeutic agents with dramatic antiretroviral activity and little toxicity at effective doses: Aromatic polycyclic diones hypericin and pseudohypericin. Proc Natl Acad Sci 85:-5230–34, 1988.

8. James JS: AIDS Treatment News #91, November 17, 1989.

9. Proceedings from The Fourth International Congress on Phytotherapy, Munich, Germany, September 10–13, 1992.

10. Chihara G, et al.: Antitumor and metastasis-inhibitory activities of lentinan as an immunomodulator: An overview. Cancer Detect Prev Suppl 1:423–43, 1987.

11. Aoki T, et al.: Low natural killer syndrome: Clinical and immunologic features. Nat Immun Cell Growth Reg 6:116–28, 1987.

12. Fujii T, et al.: Isolation and characterization of a new antitumor polysaccharide, KS-2, extracted from culture mycelia of *Lentinus edodes*. Antibiotics 31:1079–90, 1978.

13. Yamashita A, et al.: Intestinal absorption and urinary excretion of antitumor peptidomannan KS-2 after oral administration in rats. Immunopharmacol 5:209–220, 1983.

Index

Acetone, 117
Adaptogens
  and Panax ginseng, 163
  and Siberian ginseng, 159–160
Adenosine, 58
Adrenal extracts, 150
Adrenal function, 15, 143–151
  healthy function, 145–146
  nourishing adrenal glands, 147–148
  nutrient supplementation for, 148, 150
  plant-based medicines for, 150
  stress and, 144–146
  support for, 146–150
Aerobic exercise, 97
Affirmations, 53–54
AIDS patients
  St. John's wort for, 166
  T-cell ratios in, 133
  thymic hormone levels in, 131
Air pollutants, free radicals and, 66
Alarm reaction, 144
Alcohol
  free radicals and, 66
  liver function and, 119, 120
  silymarin and, 123
Allergic tension-fatigue syndrome, 32
Allergic toxemia, 32
Allergies. See also Food allergies
  adrenal extracts for, 150
  cell-mediated immunity and, 131
  thymus and, 130
  vitamin C and, 104
Aluminum, 22, 117
American Association of
  Naturopathic Physicians, 175
American Holistic Medical
  Association, 175
Amitriptyline, 167
Anatomy of an Illness (Cousins), 46
Anemia, 15, 109
Anti-EBV capsid antibody titers, 7
Antihistamines, 14
Anti-hypertensives, 14
Anti-inflammatory agents, 14
Antioxidants
  and alcohol consumption, 119, 120
  in green tea, 59
  juicing and, 65–66
  and thymus function, 138–139
Arsenic, 22
Arthritis. See Rheumatoid arthritis
Aspartate, 107–108
Asthma
  adrenal extracts for, 150
  food additives and, 83

Atherosclerosis, 137
  and hypothyroidism, 154, 155
Attitude, 48
  and CFS, 45–54
  conditioning of, 49–54
  immune system and, 135
  Siberian ginseng and, 161
Australian definition of CFS, 6
Awaken the Giant Within (Robbins), 50

Barnes, Broda, 61
Basal body temperature. See Body temperature
Basophils, 132
  mast cells, 134
B cells, 133
Benzene, 22
Beta-carotene, 64–65
  optimal level for, 99–100
Betaine, 121
Bicycling, 97
Birth control pills, 14
Black tea, 58–59
Blood sugar levels, 38
Blood tests
  for CFS, 16–17
  for food allergies, 35
B-lymphocytes, 131
Body temperature, 35–36
  fasting and, 126
  thyroid extracts, use of, 156
Bodywork, 93–95
Boredom and CFS, 47
Borrelia bugdorferi, 9
Bowel tolerance of vitamin C, 105
Breads in Healthy Exchange System, 75–76
Breakfast menus, 82
Breathing, 92
Brekhman, I. I., 160
Brucella, 9

Cadmium, 22, 117
Caffeine, 56–59
  in green tea, 59
Caloric needs, 67
Camellia sinensis, 58–59
Cancer
  as cause of CFS, 14
  cell-mediated immunity and, 131
  fruit and, 64
  green tea and, 59
  interferon in therapy for, 10
  lentinan and, 168–169
  mushroom extracts and, 168